D

Kettlebell Conditioning

1

The Body Coach®

Kettlebell Conditioning

4-Phase BodyBell® Training System
with Australia's Body Coach®

Plus 25 Bonus Medicine Ball Training Drills

Paul Collins

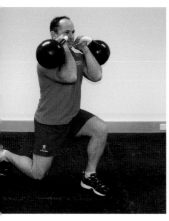 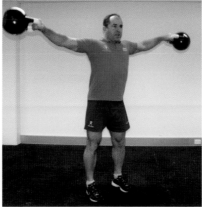 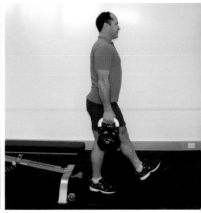

Meyer & Meyer Sport

British Library Cataloguing in Publication Data
A catalogue record for this book is available from the British Library

Kettlebell Conditioning
Maidenhead: Meyer & Meyer Sport (UK) Ltd., 2011
ISBN 978-1-84126-316-8

© 2011 Paul Collins (text & photos)
and Meyer & Meyer Sport (UK) Ltd. (Layout)
2nd Edition 2012
Auckland, Beirut, Budapest, Cairo, Cape Town, Dubai, Indianapolis,
Kindberg, Maidenhead, Sydney, Olten, Singapore, Tehran, Toronto
Member of the World
Sport Publishers' Association (WSPA)
www.w-s-p-a.org
Printed and bound by: B.O.S.S Druck und Medien GmbH, Germany
ISBN 978-1-84126-316-8
E-Mail: info@m-m-sports.com
www.m-m-sports.com

Contents

Trademarks
Body Coach®, The Body Coach®, Fastfeet®, Quickfeet®, Speedhoop®, Posturefit®, Spinal Unloading Block®, 3 Hour Rule®, BodyBell®, Australia's Personal Trainer™, Speed for Sport™, Collins-Technique™, Coach Collins™, Collins Lateral Fly™, 20-40-60 Exercise Principle™, Core-in Motion Method™ (CIMM™), Abdominal Wheel System™, GTS™ Grid Training System™, and 3Bs Principle™, Collins Pivot Technique™, Body Coach Zone™, The Stretching Zone™, The Flexibility Zone™, The Posture Zone™, The Yoga Zone™, The Pilates Zone™, The Strength Zone™, The Aerobic Zone™, The Core Zone™, The Speed Zone™, The Recovery Zone™, The Workout Zone™, The Training Zone™ are trademarks of Paul Collins.

About the Author

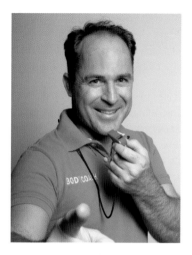

Paul Collins, Australia's Personal Trainer™, is founder of The Body Coach® fitness products, books, DVDs and educational coaching systems, which help people to get fit, lose weight, look good and feel great. Coaching since age 14, Paul has personally trained world-class athletes and teams in a variety of sports from track and field, squash, rugby, golf, soccer and tennis, to members of the Australian World Championship Karate Team, Manly 1st Grade Rugby Union Team and members of the world-renowned Australian Olympic and Paralympic Swimming teams. Paul is an outstanding athlete in his own right. He has played grade rugby league in the national competition, and has been an A-grade squash player, National Budokan Karate Champion, and NSW State Masters Athletics Track & Field Champion.

A recipient of the prestigious Fitness Instructor of the Year Award in Australia, Paul is regarded by his peers as the "Trainers' Trainer" having educated thousands of fitness instructors and personal trainers, as well as appearing in TV, radio and print media internationally. Over the past decade, Paul has presented to various national sporting bodies, including the Australian Track & Field Coaching Association, Australia Swimming Coaches and Teachers Association, Australian Rugby League, Australian Karate Federation, and the Australian Fitness Industry. He has also traveled in order to present a highly entertaining series of corporate health & well-being seminars for companies focused on developing a Body for Success™ in life and in business.

Paul holds a bachelor's degree in physical education from the Australian College of Physical Education. He is also a certified trainer and assessor, and strength and conditioning coach with the Australian Sports Commission and Olympic Weightlifting Club Power Coach with the Australian Weightlifting Federation. As a certified personal trainer with Fitness Australia, Paul possesses over two decades of experience as a talented athlete, coach and mentor for people of all age groups and ability levels seeking to achieve their optimal potential.

In his free time, Paul enjoys traveling, adventures, food, restaurants, movies, and competing in track and field. He resides in Sydney, Australia.

For more details, visit: www.thebodycoach.com

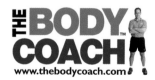

A Word from the Body Coach®

Welcome! I'm the Body Coach® Paul Collins, Australia's Personal Trainer™, and I'm here to guide you through Kettlebell (KB) Conditioning. Founded in Russia, kettlebells are heavy cast iron balls with a handle that come in a number of weights. They are used as a training tool to develop a lean, strong athletic physique.

The unique shape of the kettlebell challenges the whole body as the hand, arm, shoulder and core region controls the displacement of weight and counteraction of muscles with each movement. Exercises progress from single, static, isolated movements to more dynamic functional drills and double KB exercises, which are excellent for improving athletic performance. With this in mind, I have developed the 4-Phase BodyBell® Training System™ to provide you with a method of progressive development training for the whole body using kettlebells. The BodyBell® System helps steer you through essential foundational exercises, key movements and swing patterns prior to taking on more complex power drills using both single and double kettlebells with over possible 100 drills.

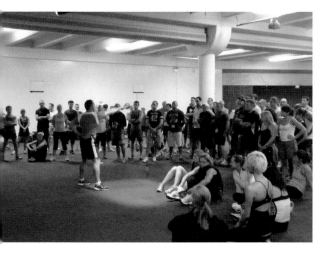

This book is part of The Body Coach® Book Series, designed to support your favorite exercise products and fitness pursuits by making exercise easy to understand and implement by showing you what to do and how to do it in simple terms for a better learning experience and greater results, thus ensuring you are guided all the way!

Paul presenting at International Filex Convention, Sydney, Australia

I look forward to working with you!

Paul Collins
The Body Coach®
Australia's Personal Trainer™

CHAPTER 1
Kettlebell Training

What is a Kettlebell (KB)?

Kettlebells, which originated in Russia, are heavy cast iron balls with a handle that are used by athletes for functional strength development and by fitness enthusiasts for training variety. The design of the kettlebell makes it unique because when you grip the handle, the weight is displaced differently when compared to that of a KB. This weight displacement makes you work harder to control the movement by counterbalancing and control the handle by gripping it at different angles of movement. The size and shape of the kettlebell varies (depending on the manufacturer) in handle shape, thickness and bell density and size, which in turn challenges the body and technique requirements in many ways. Sizes start from around 4kg (8 pounds) and increase in 4kg increments with beginners using 4kg–16kg KB and more advanced athletes using KBs that are 20kg to 60kg or more

Benefits of Kettlebell Training

Kettlebell training aims to develop strength through all planes of movement. Because the kettlebell aligns with the body's center of gravity, the athlete must work harder to balance and stabilize the weight throughout all movement patterns. This requires a strong contribution from the muscles of the arm, shoulder and core region. Along with this comes improvement in strength, power and body awareness for better muscle control by addressing both acceleration and deceleration of movement. Best of all, the challenging nature of kettlebell training works the whole body, making exercise fun and rewarding!

4-Stage BodyBell® Training System™

Every good exercise program starts with a method by which training principles are based upon. In my book *Awesome Abs*, I devised a 5-Phase Abdominal Training System for maximizing your core potential. In *Speed for Sport*™, I devised a 6-Stage Fastfeet® Training Model for maximizing your speed potential. In *Functional Fitness*, I devised a functional fitness method (FFM) with 6 Key Movement Patterns that aim to provide a balance of muscular strength, fitness and mobility throughout multiple planes of motion. In *Strength Training for Men*, I devised the 5-Phase Core-Strength to Power Conversion Training System™, which aims to improve the fundamental core-strength, mobility and coordination required for Olympic lifting and power gains. In *Core-Fitness*, I introduced a new approach focused on cavity-based training along with the Core-in-Motion Method™ for improved muscular control in functional athletic positions. In *Athletic Abs*, I introduced the Top 10 abdominal exercises of all time using the revolutionary Abdominal Wheel System™. In *Dynamic Dumbbell Training*, I introduced a 3-Stage Dynamic Dumbbell Training System™ that progresses the practitioner through stages of strength, function and power training. And now, in this book, I have developed the 4-Stage BodyBell® Training System™ that allows you to learn the basic strength and swing pattern drills before tackling more complex power-orientated movement patterns.

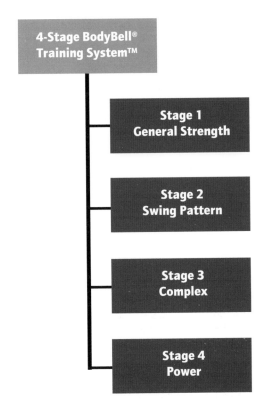

4-Stage BodyBell® Progression

In any training program, a method of progression first needs to be established so that one knows where he is starting and where he needs to progress to. The innovative 4-Stage BodyBell® progression applied here allows you time to establish appropriate strength throughout the body, in your muscles, joints, energy and nervous systems so that you can progressively adapt to new functional and more powerful swings and movement patterns over time for optimal athletic gains.

Stage 1: General Strength

The general strength preparation phase is based on a diverse range of strength movement exercises using kettlebells that aim to improve muscle coordination and endurance, neural adaptation and body awareness. The main exercises provided in Stage 1 involve individual isolated exercises, as well as compound movement exercises that target multiple muscle groups. This stage includes exercise instruction in technique and breathing for increasing body awareness and maximizing muscular strength, endurance and kettlebell control.

Stage 2: Swing Pattern

The swing pattern provides the foundation for ongoing kettlebell development. Swing movements are distinctive drills that separate kettlebell training from any other strength-based exercises. Correct technique and technical progressions allow the body to increase neuromuscular firing patterns, which improves strength, coordination and timing throughout the whole body.

Stage 3: Complex Kettlebell Exercises

As one improves general strength and masters the swing pattern, this stage provides the foundation for more complex, functional-based exercises to be performed, which further challenges strength, timing and neuromuscular coordination. Due to the complexity and muscular counterbalance required to control each movement, the aim is to start light and build muscular endurance before increasing the kettlebell weight. As movement function and control improve, the kettlebell weight is increased, as well as the repetitions (or time) and sets to heighten the challenge, with quality of movement (over quantity) the main objective at all times.

Stage 4: Power Development

After improving general strength and mastering the swing patterns and more complex kettlebell exercises, your body will have developed the essential core strength, coordination and timing (in addition to rewiring the strength of the neuromuscular framework throughout the body) for more advanced, full-body power-based technical drills. In Stage 4, we concentrate on exercises that link two or more strength foundation exercises together to form a part or sequence of a simulated Olympic-lifting style movement using kettlebells, which generates a high level of speed, force and power. The objective here is to never sacrifice lifting technique for a heavier KB weight and to ensure that strength and functional movement patterns are in place prior to implementation in Stage 4. This is essential for building correct technique, muscular coordination and developing the timing of more powerful lifts along with the continual adaptation of the neuromuscular framework as part of a power progression using submaximal KB loads for mastering technique before increasing KB loads.

Applying the 3Bs Principle™

Every exercise has a number of key elements to consider when setting up and performing a movement. Applying correct technique from the onset will help establish good form, which is ultimately maintained until the repetitions or set is completed. The key elements required in order to maintain good body position while exercising form part of a simple exercise set-up phrase that I've termed the **3Bs Principle™**, which is outlined as follows:

1. Brace

Activating and bracing your abdominal (core) muscles while exercising is important because it helps increase awareness of your body position while also helping to unload any stress placed on the lower back region.

2. Breath

In foundation and core-strength training, you **breathe out** when you exert force, such as pushing the KB overhead in the shoulder press exercise or the body rising up straight from a squat position. You then **breathe in** with recovery, such as lowering the KB back down from overhead or lowering the body and bending the legs when performing a squat. In other exercises, such as Stage 2 Swing Patterns or more complex movement patterns, breathing should remain deep and constant at all times throughout each exercise. If unsure, just ensure that your breathing remains constant, in general – breathing out when you exert a force and breathing in upon recovery. Never hold your breath.

3. Body Position

To complete the 3Bs Principle™, the third B relates to one's ability to maintain good body position and technique with each exercise. In all exercises, ensure good head, neck, spine and pelvic alignment is maintained at all times. The overall focus of each exercise should be on the quality of the movement at all times.

The next time you perform any exercise, simply apply the 3Bs Principle™ from start to finish in order to maintain correct technique and body posture, which will help maximize your strength and power gains.

Functional Warm-up

As the scientific knowledge and understanding of our body and training practices improve, it seems a functional (or dynamic) warm-up plays a number of crucial roles toward improving quality of movement and athletic performance in the following ways:

- Gradually increase your heart rate and core body temperature by performing activities on the move
- Set your muscular and nervous systems in motion
- Work muscles and joints through an appropriate range of movement
- Heighten the ability of your muscles to contract and be ready for the activities that follow in order to reduce the risk of injury
- Allow you to warm up your muscles so that they are ready to work at full speed
- Improves physical and mental alertness by setting the tone for the rest of the session
- Incorporates a routine of exercises that improve balance, technique and coordination
- Improves athleticism through establishing good technique and range of motion

Muscles that are warm and without movement restriction ensure the quality of movement found in the strength training exercises that follow. This is maximized when applying the 3Bs Principle™ with each exercise as it ensures good body posture while helping maximize strength, functional and power gains.

Warm-up Progression

The first stage of a good warm-up is increasing the heart rate and muscle temperature through cardiovascular movement, such as walking or light jogging, or using a stationary bike or rowing machine, treadmill or similar apparatus for approximately 5-10 minutes. This also helps focus one's mind on the exercise program that follows.

The second stage focuses on range of movement and control of each joint. This is achieved by combining a dynamic movement through a range of motion followed by brief stretching or a series of stretches while the muscle is warm, except where a joint is hypermobile and a stability approach is required (no stretching) for better muscle control. During this period, you can also gauge whether specific muscles require further stretching or muscle control techniques. This pattern is demonstrated below as part of the Coach Collins™ Warm-up Sequence. (For more information, refer also to The Body Coach Speed for Sport™ book.)

Coach Collins™ Warm-up Sequence – Cycle 1

Instructions:
Complete the following warm-up sequence from 1-8 before repeating drills on opposite leg for a total of 16 movements for 6 seconds each *(approximately 3 minute dynamic warm-up stretching sequence).*

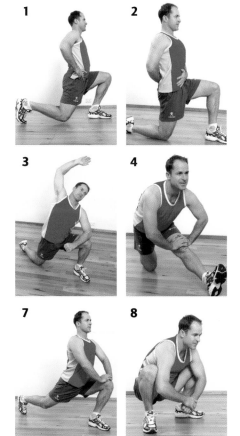
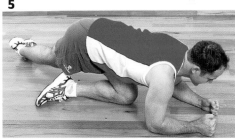
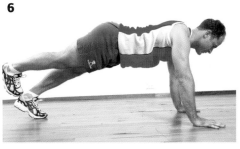

1. Start by performing 6 x stationary lunges with left leg forward rising up and down.
2. Lower rear knee to ground and tilt pelvis forward to stretch rear thigh for 6 seconds.
3. Lower left forearm onto front thigh whilst extending right arm overhead and leaning the body across to the left side for 6 seconds.
4. Lean body back and straighten front leg whilst placing hands on thigh to support lower back and stretch the hamstrings for 6 seconds.
5. Bend the front leg and rest across shin whilst taking rear leg across body and resting on forearms and stretching the hip and gluteal regions for 6 seconds.
6. Raise onto both hands in a front support position and rest the right foot on the heel of the left foot and stretch the calves for 3 seconds before performing a few light bounces for 3 seconds.
7. Step the left leg forwards and place both hands on front thigh keeping torso long and tall whilst stretching for 6 seconds.
8. Step forward with feet shoulder-width apart, with arms inside knee whilst pushing knees out for 6 seconds to stretch the adductors.

Coach Collins™ Warm-up Sequence – Cycle 2

The kettlebell can also be used as part of the warm-up cycle. Using a light pair of kettlebells, perform the following exercise sequence in a continuous manner before moving onto the next exercise without resting! This is meant to warm up the muscles, tendons and joints of the upper body for more demanding exercises, as well as bring focus and attention to establishing good body position. Any muscular tension or restriction felt at this stage needs to be addressed prior to further training.

1. Perform 8 front raises (Page 47)
2. Perform 8 lateral raises (Page 56)
3. Perform 8 upright rows (Page 43)
4. Perform 8 bent over rows (Page 38)
5. Perform 8 overhead presses (Page 54)
6. Perform 8 biceps curls (Page 66)
7. Perform 8 triceps extensions (Page 61)

Coach Collins™ Warm-up Sequence – Cycle 3

Cycle 3 of the warm-up phase aims to warm up the muscles, tendons and joints of the lower body. Using a light pair of kettlebells, perform the following exercise sequence before moving onto the next exercise without resting!

1. Perform 8 alternate leg forward lunges (Page 77)
2. Perform 8 front squats (Page 84)
3. Perform 8 alternate leg side lunges (Page 77)
4. Perform 8 push-presses (Page 18)
5. Perform 8 hip thrusts (Page 18)

Prior to entering the main phase of your training, it should be remembered that a light to moderate KB should be used as a warm-up set prior to each exercise. This enables you bring focus and attention to each exercise, as well as the more demanding KB weight that will soon follow.

Progressive Resistance Training

In any physical activity, your muscles grow in response to the challenge placed upon them. Over time, the muscles adapt to this stimulus and require an additional challenge for muscular strength gains to occur. The stimulus for this change revolves around **8 Key Elements,** some of which work simultaneously.

8 Key Elements	Description
1. Exercise intensity	Weight (or mass) being lifted; based upon a percentage of one's maximum lift or 1RM (repetition maximum) used by advanced athletes and coaches for establishing training loads, reps and sets
2. Speed of movement – repetition ratio	Speed ratio of concentric and eccentric movement as well as mass being lifted – i.e. slow, fast or a combination of both, for example - 3:1:1 Ratio (or 3 seconds eccentric, 1 second transition, 1 second concentric) used in hypertrophy. Variations of these ratios apply, which can manipulate the intensity and max-strength gains
3. Time muscle is under tension	Number of repetitions being performed; speed of movement and the exercise intensity
4. Type of exercise	Actual exercise and movement being performed for specific muscle group – as there are many variations for each muscle group
5. Volume of work	Total number of repetitions and sets being performed as well as the frequency
6. Rest periods	Recovery period between exercises and sets can dictate fatigue or regeneration
7. Frequency	How often you train each week
8. Mental focus	How much effort and focus you put into your training session

In strength training, using kettlebells and variations of these 8 Key Elements plays a major role in establishing your training goals and reaching your specific outcomes.

Safety Tips

Avoid Overuse

When isolating specific muscles, be careful not to create an unbalanced condition. Unbalanced muscles may allow a particular muscle to work harder than the supporting and stabilizing muscles, thereby increasing the chances of injury. The aim is to create muscular balance by working all muscle groups as opposed to focusing on any single area. Ensure full range of motion is available without any undue stress.

No-Pain Principle

If, when exercising, you feel any sharp or concerning pain, always stop the exercise immediately. Be sure to perform a proper warm-up before continuing. If pain persists, always seek medical advice right away.

Kettlebell Variations

Different kettlebell brands will vary in shape, weight, size and handle thickness. This is important to remember as it will often change the weight displacement and movement mechanics, thus requiring a higher skill focus.

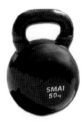

Choosing a Kettlebell Weight

When starting any new exercise or movement pattern, the kettlebell weight should be light and the technique mastered before progressing to a heavier weight. This ensures the muscles, joints and connective tissues have adapted to the demands of each exercise. Kettlebells start at 4-kilograms (kg) or 8.8-pounds and progress in 4kg increments up to 40kg, and then 50kg or heavier. In most instances, people start with a 4kg-16kg kettlebell in order to learn the basics of each exercise and gain proficiency before progressing to a heavier kettlebell.

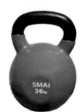

Static Strength Before Dynamic Strength

With kettlebells, it is very important to start with basic, isolated movement patterns to build good core strength and body awareness before introducing more dynamic, functional multi-muscle or complex movement patterns. In other words, learn and perform simple movements before moving onto complex ones.

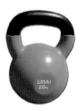

Hand Control

In most exercises, as the exercise movement occurs, it requires actions where the handle itself swivels within the palm of the hand before a firm grip is applied. This requires good hand, wrist, elbow, arm and shoulder strength for movement control and essential core strength to maintain balance.

Speed of Movement

The speed of movement at which each repetition is performed plays a vital role in kettlebell training. Due to the weight displacement, movements need to first be learned in a slow, controlled pattern using a light kettlebell to secure essential muscle memory that can be drawn upon when advancing to more dynamic movements of a similar nature using a heavier kettlebell.

Loss of Form: If form is lost while performing any exercise repetition or set, the movement should be stopped or readjusted applying the 3Bs Principle™. Remember, kettlebell training is all about quality of movement at all times!

Coach: The unique nature of the kettlebell requires a qualified coach or personal trainer to demonstrate and assess your exercise technique with each exercise.

Check the Product: If the kettlebell is damaged and/or has any sharp metal edges, discontinue use and replace the product immediately. Always follow the manufacturer's instructions and guidelines.

Open Space: Be sure when working out with the kettlebell that you are in a clear, open space. For example, a 3 meter x 3 meter area is good.

Central Nervous System (CNS): The heavier the kettlebell and the quicker the movement, the higher the demand on the central nervous system. This leads to rapid fatigue and must be controlled with high quality, short interval exercise periods, and maintaining good form, followed by longer rest periods inbetween sets that allow full recovery.

Cooling Down After Exercise

The practice of cooling down gradually after exercise for 5 minutes or so with gentle exercise followed by stretching plays an important role in helping your heart rate and breathing to return to normal. As a general rule, allow 5-10 minutes of post-exercise stretching for every one hour of exercise. Make these post-exercise stretches more thorough than your warm-up stretches. Be sure you stretch all the major muscle groups you used during your exercise session. Stretch each muscle group for 10 to 20 seconds or more, 2 to 3 times. For examples of stretches to perform, refer to *The Body Coach Stretching Book*.

CHAPTER 2
Body Bell® Training System™:

7 Key Kettlebell Movement Patterns

1. Hip Thrust Development

The hip thrust plays a major role in the kettlebell swing motion of the arms and movement of the legs in a squat motion while exerting pelvic control of the lower body region. In order to learn the required technique of swinging the hips forward and tightening the glutes while preventing the legs from performing any swinging motions, the following three exercises should be mastered before any swinging movement is introduced.

1A: Hamstring bridge with pelvic thrust and glute tightening

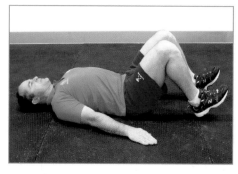

Lowered

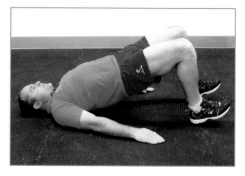

Pelvic thrust & glute tightening

Lying on your back, squeeze your glutes and tighten your abs as you rise up onto your heels. Exhale during exertion.

1B: Sumo Squat

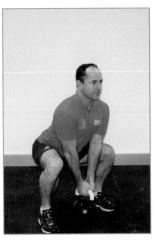
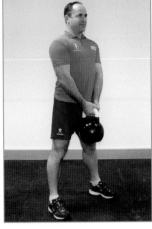

Start

Raise, thrust and glute tightening

Description

- Start with feet wider than shoulder-width, arms extended down, gripping KB, which is resting on the ground
- Exhale upward
- Push hips forward and squeeze (tighten) butt cheeks
- Push feet into the ground
- Ensure core is tight
- Inhale while lowering

1C: Standing Hip Thrust (Counterbalance Mechanism)

Restrain your core by squeezing your glutes and tightening your abs when swinging the KB up from a squat position with the arms while locking the legs out. Practice first without the KB by just swinging your hands in front of your body. Next, introduce a light KB in both hands and practice as shown below.

All movements utilizing a kettlebell require counterbalancing throughout the body for movement control. For instance, while swinging the kettlebell upward with the arms and extending the hips forward, the movement requires counterbalancing throughout the posterior muscles of the calf, hamstrings, gluteal and lower back regions. As the body extends, the hips are quickly snapped forward while the gluteal muscles are squeezed together. Avoid leaning backwards.

As the kettlebell swings back down between the legs, the abdominal core muscles need to be heavily contracted as an effective counterbalance mechanism.

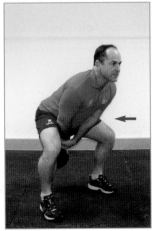
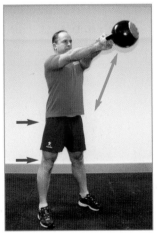

Timing and proficiency between muscle groups in each movement is the vital ingredient for successful kettlebell training. Start with a light kettlebell and master this movement before progressing to a heavier kettlebell.

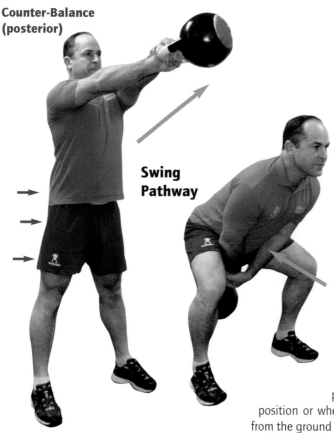

Counter-Balance (posterior)

Swing Pathway

Counterbalance Mechanism Overview

As the kettlebell pathway of the arms rises up in front of the body, the counterbalance occurs through the posterior (rear) side of the body (in the back and gluteal muscles). In the other hand, in the lowering phase of the swing (and squat), the counterbalance occurs through the bracing of the abdominal muscles.

Counter-Balance (Anterior) Abdominal muscles

2. The Rack Position

The rack position refers to the position of the arm in a starting position or when the kettlebell is raised to the chest from the ground and prior to overhead lifting.

Variables of the rack position include an overhand grip in the following positions:

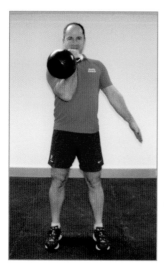

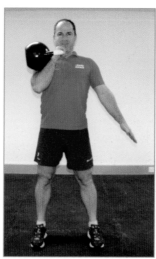

Deciding which two rack positions to use will depend on one's flexibility and muscle control. Be sure the shoulders, back and shoulder blades are squeezed together. Abdominals should be braced using the 3Bs Principle™.

1. Palms to chest   *2. Knuckles to side*

3. Pick-up Position

3A: Starting Point

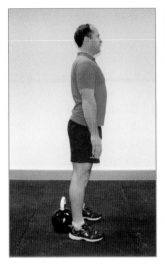
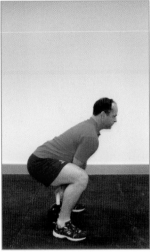

Step in front of the KB (behind heels), squat down, reach the arms through the legs, and grasp the handle with both hands, knuckles forward.

Note: Ensure you have established a flat back position. Rounding of the back can occur from limited hamstrings flexibility in the squat position which needs to be addressed through regular stretching and mobility of the hamstrings, gluteal and hip regions for movement efficiency to occur.

3B: Alternate Exercise

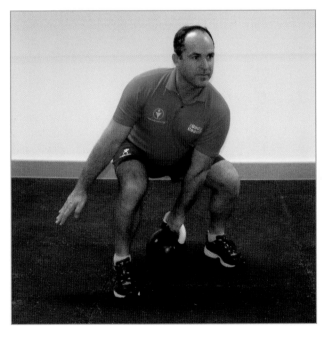

With a single hand, pick up the KB with knuckles inward, thumb backwards.

4. Overhead Grip Positions

Below are a few of the main grip positions possible with various overhead movement patterns. Variations of these grip positions can be applied using single or double KBs. Ensure quality of motion and safety at all times.

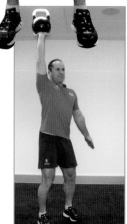

Knuckles backwards

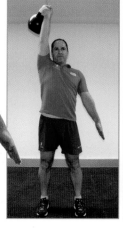

Knuckles to side

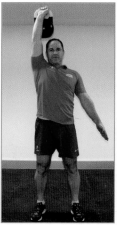

Bottom-up position – holding handle

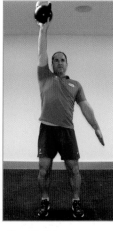

Fingertip Press – under base on KB

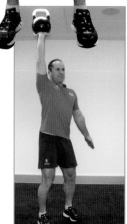

Waiter Press – palm under KB

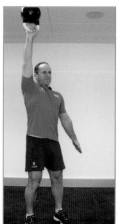

Double Waiter Press – palm under KB

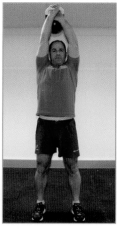

Grip Through – two hands on single KB with underhand grip

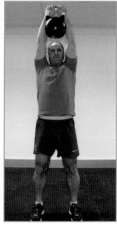

Grip Through – two hands on single KB with overhand grip and thumb around handle

Note: Additional arm movements can also be performed in squat and lunge positions.

5. Back Position and Angles

The depth and angle at which one lowers the body, in terms of leg bend (squat) and body angle from hip to head (specifically in any swing motion), determines the load placed on specific regions of the body, as shown below.

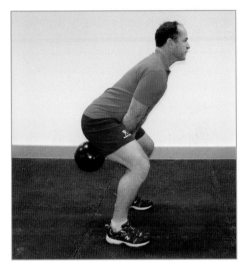

Gluteal and hamstrings emphasis

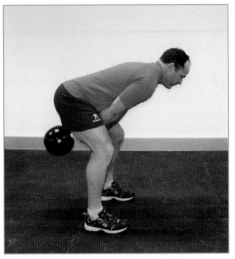

Lower back emphasis (not recommended)

Variations
- Glute emphasis
- Squat depth and leg angle(s)

Hand Positions:
- Single arm swing
- Double hand swing ⎬ Hand Angle
- Balance arm (resting or raised)
- Knuckles forward
- Knuckles inward

6. Swing Arc Range 1-4

The swing arc ranges of the kettlebell in any single or double arm swing motion in front of the body determines the concentric and eccentric transition loading points of the arm, shoulder, and back muscles, as well as the application of the counterbalance mechanism. As a result, it is important to ensure that a good range of motion and muscle control is first achieved through light loading endurance swing patterns. This helps establish good body awareness, muscle control, strength and endurance, correct firing patterns and movement efficiency throughout the whole body. Thus, whether using a single arm or both hands, be sure to establish a strong foundation over a 6-8 week period using lighter kettlebells and a gradual increase in swing arc range of motion 1–3 to establish and maintain control. Avoid going higher than arc level 3 unless under the guidance of a certified strength and conditioning coach.

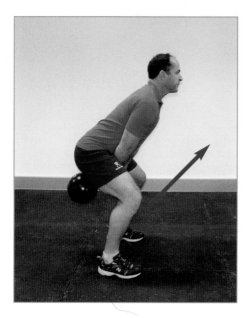 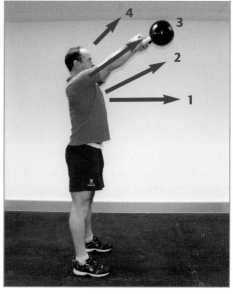

Ensure swing control and body awareness by maintaining the 3Bs Principle™.

Breathing Pattern
- Exhale – up
- Inhale – down

7. The Quick Snap

Once you have progressed through the first six key kettlebell patterns, you will be ready for an important movement transition I've termed the Quick Snap. In simple terms, the Quick Snap applies to achieving the most fluid movement from the ground or any single arm swing motion into the rack position with the greatest speed and control.

By gripping the kettlebell in one hand, knuckles inward, thumbs backwards from the ground position (as shown previously with left hand in 3B) or while swinging the KB between your legs for an upcoming transition, provides one of the most efficient starting points from which this transition into the rack position can occur. With the thumb pointing backwards, the wrist and forearm are positioned perfectly for a quick, efficient and controlled transition into the rack position, with the KB rotating around the hand reducing the load placed on the wrist and forearm in the rack position. As many similar transitions occur each time in training, the ability to better control such movements will help reduce the risk of injury and forearm bruising that may occur using poor transition technique. For this reason, start light and practice the Quick Snap using each hand.

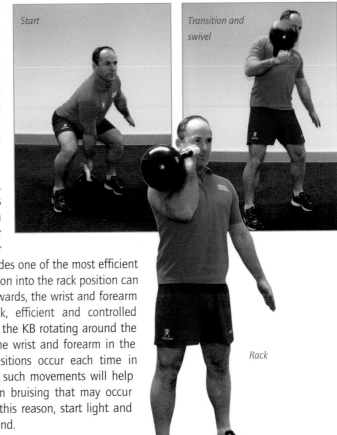

Start

Transition and swivel

Rack

Five Essential KB Training Safety Tips

1. Establish a KB workout zone – a large, free-swing area
2. Start with a lighter KB and gradually increase KB weight as muscle control, foundational strength, and endurance improve
3. Apply the 3Bs Principle™ for constant awareness throughout each pattern
4. Always focus on quality of movement over quantity!
5. Include appropriate rest periods for maximal strength and power gains, and to avoid any susceptibility to injury due to overuse

With these 7 key movement patterns and essential KB training safety tips in mind, let's get started with Stage 1 of the BodyBell® Training System.

CHAPTER 3
Stage 1: General Kettlebell Strength Exercises

General kettlebell strength exercises provide a key foundation for improving the strength, endurance, muscle control and body awareness required before undertaking more complex KB power drills. In Stage 1, the objective is to develop a solid foundation of strength, endurance, coordination and timing by focusing on enhancing one's muscular framework and neuromuscular control using a KB in various planes of motion.

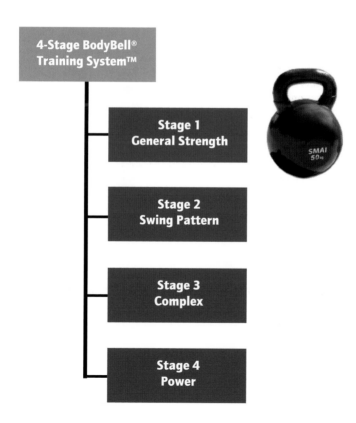

**4-Stage BodyBell®
Training System™**

**Stage 1
General Strength**

**Stage 2
Swing Pattern**

**Stage 3
Complex**

**Stage 4
Power**

This chapter focuses on key exercises meant to improve muscular gains throughout the body. Exercises include both isolated, single joint and compound, multi-joint exercises in the following muscle regions:

- Chest
- Back
- Arms
  - Triceps
  - Biceps
- Shoulders
- Legs
  - Deadlifts this is not a muscle region
  - Lunges this is not a muscle region
  - Squats this is not a muscle region
- Calves
- Abs & Core

CHEST

Strengthening the chest and arms in unison with the abdominal region plays a major role in body balance between the upper and lower body. The basic rule for all chest exercises is the narrower the hand position and movement, the greater the triceps contribution and the lesser the chest contribution; conversely, the wider the hand or movement angle position, the greater the chest contribution and the lesser the triceps contribution. The primary and secondary muscles targeted are:

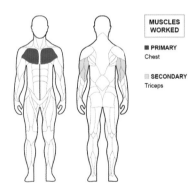

MUSCLES WORKED

■ PRIMARY
Chest

▨ SECONDARY
Triceps

- **Pectoralis (Chest)** – Large fan-shaped muscle that covers the front of the upper chest.

- **Triceps** – The rear side of the upper arm.

8. Single Arm Chest Press

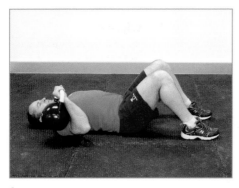

Start

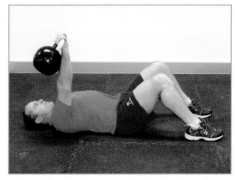

Mid-point

Description
- Lie on ground with knees and arm bent, gripping the KB in one hand, knuckles facing backwards and the other arm resting by your side
- Apply the 3Bs Principle™
- While exhaling, push the KB straight up vertically until your arm is locked above your chest before lowering in a controlled manner
- Repeat drill with opposite arm

Exercise Variations
- Lying on the ground
- Lying on a flat weight bench
- Lying on a Bosu® ball
- Lying on a foam roller
- Lying on a fitness ball – requires body rotation and shoulder raise with arm extension

Exercise Variation: Rotate body with arm raises

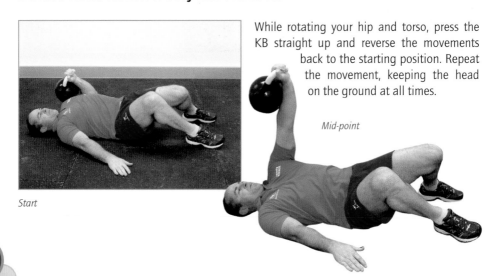

Start

While rotating your hip and torso, press the KB straight up and reverse the movements back to the starting position. Repeat the movement, keeping the head on the ground at all times.

Mid-point

9. Two-handed floor press

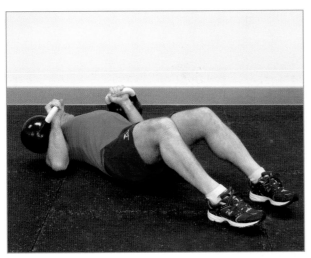

Start

Description
- Lie on ground with knees and arms bent down by side, gripping KBs in both hands, knuckles facing backwards
- Apply the 3Bs Principle™
- While breathing out, simultaneously push both arms straight up vertically until they are locked above your chest, then lower them in a controlled movement

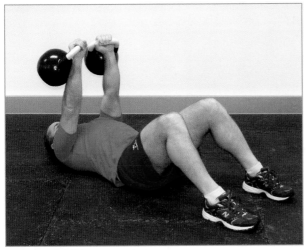

Mid-point

Be sure the KB is pressed straight up, avoiding any forward or backward movement behind the shoulders.

10. KB Alternating Chest Press

Description
- Lie on the ground with knees and arms bent down by your side, gripping KBs in both hands, knuckles facing backwards
- Apply the 3Bs Principle™
- While exhaling, push one arm straight up, lifting the rear side of your shoulder off the ground by rotating your hip and torso until your arm is locked vertically above your chest
- Lower your arm in a controlled motion and repeat with opposite arm

Be sure the KB is pressed straight up, avoiding any forward or backward movement behind the shoulders.

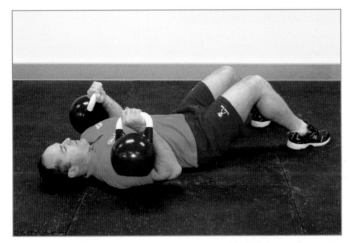

Start

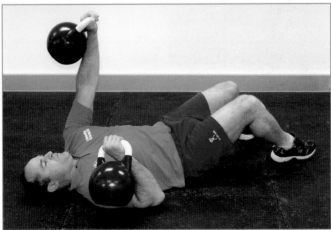

Mid-point

11. Flat Bench Press

Description
- Lie on your back on a flat weight bench with your feet resting on the ground shoulder-width apart for support. Both arms are extended vertically, holding KBs with palms facing up and the hands close together
- Apply the 3Bs Principle™
- Inhale as you simultaneously lower both arms by bending the elbows until the KBs are level with your chest
- Exhale as you raise the KBs back up to the starting position to complete one repetition

Variations
This exercise can also be performed lying on a fitness ball or incline bench in order to challenge different areas of the chest.

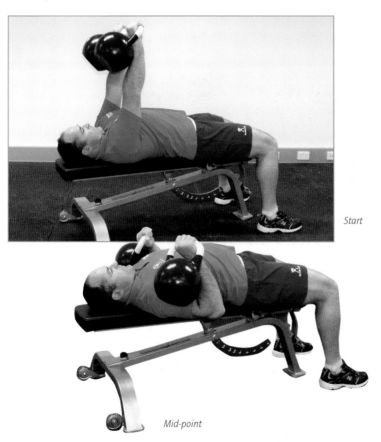

Start

Mid-point

12. Alternate Flat Bench Press 2+1

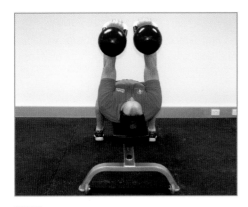

START

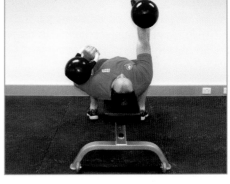

Lower left arm

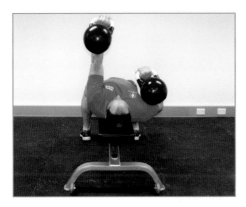

Lower right arm

Description

- Lie on your back on a flat weight bench with your feet resting on the ground shoulder-width apart for support. Both arms are extended vertically, holding the KBs with palms facing up and hands close together
- Apply the 3Bs Principle™
- Inhale as you lower one KB by bending the elbow until the KB is level with your chest, while ensuring your core is held strong

- Exhale as you alternate the arm movement, simultaneously raising the lowered KB back up vertically and lowering the other KB down to your chest to complete one repetition

Variations

This exercise can be performed by lowering and raising one arm before repeating with the other, as well as on an incline bench or fitness ball.

13. Chest Fly

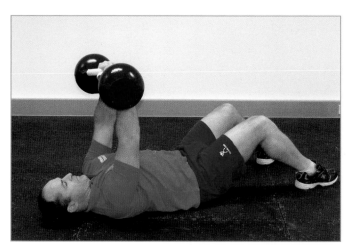

Start

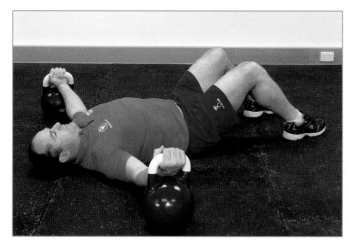

Mid-point

Description

- Lie on your back on the ground with knees bent and arm raised vertically above your chest gripping KBs in both hands held close, with the arms slightly bent and knuckles facing outward
- Apply the 3Bs Principle™
- Inhale as you simultaneously lower both arms in a semicircular motion, keeping the arms in a fixed position, until the KBs reach the ground. Be sure the lower back does not arch
- Exhale as you raise both KBs simultaneously back up to the starting position to complete one repetition

Note: This exercise can also be performed on a fitness ball, flat bench, incline bench or decline bench in order to challenge different areas of the chest.

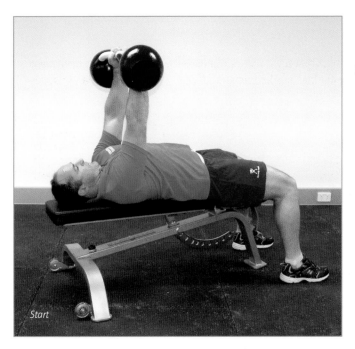

Start

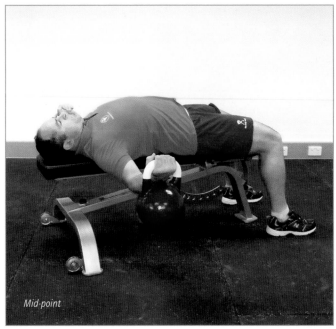

Mid-point

14. Flat Bench Fly

Description

- Lie on your back on a flat weight bench with your feet resting on the ground shoulder-width apart for support, and both arms extended vertically above the chest gripping KBs in both hands, which are held close, with the arms slightly bent and knuckles facing outward

- Apply the 3Bs Principle™

- Inhale as you simultaneously lower both arms in a semicircular motion, keeping the arms in a fixed position, until KBs reach the ground. Be sure your lower back does not arch

- Exhale as you raise both KBs simultaneously back up to the starting position to complete one repetition

Note: This exercise can also be performed on a fitness ball, incline bench or decline bench to challenge different areas of the chest.

BACK

The following exercises target both the back and arm muscles. Exercises include movement through the shoulder blades, shoulder girdle, elbow and wrist joints. The primary muscles used include:

- **Trapezius –** Upper portion of the back, sometimes referred to as "traps" (upper trapezius), this is the muscle running from the back of the neck to the shoulder.

- **Latissimus dorsi –** Large muscles of the mid-back. When properly trained, they give the back a nice V shape, making the waist appear smaller. Exercise examples include pull-ups, chin-ups and pull downs.

- **Deltoids –** The cap of the shoulder. This muscle has three parts, anterior deltoid (the front), medial deltoid (the middle), and posterior deltoid (the rear). Different movements target the different parts.

- **Rhomboids –** Muscles in the middle of the upper back between the shoulder blades. They're worked during chin-ups and other moves that bring the shoulder blades together.

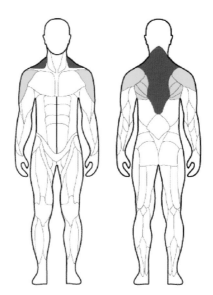

MUSCLES WORKED

■ **PRIMARY**
Upper Back

☐ **SECONDARY**
Shoulders

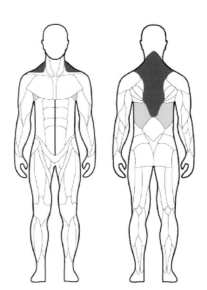

MUSCLES WORKED

■ **PRIMARY**
Upper Back

☐ **SECONDARY**
Mid Back

15. Single Arm Row

Description

- Stand with one leg forward and the other back
- Rest forward hand above knee with rear arm extended down by the front foot – knuckles out
- Apply the 3 Bs Principle™
- Keeping the wrist straight, raise arm up high by your side leading with the elbow, then lower
- Repeat drill with opposite arm

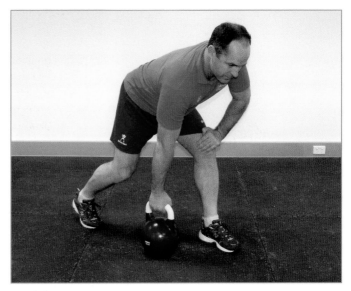

Start

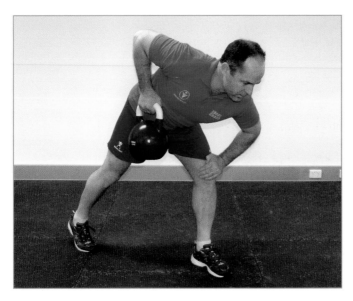

Mid-point

16. Lineman Row

![Start photo]

Start

Description
- Stand tall with feet wider than shoulder-width apart while gripping a single KB at arm's length in front of your body
- Bend at the hip and knee while leaning the torso forward until almost parallel to the ground. Keep the arm at ankle level with knuckles facing outward and the opposite hand resting on your knee
- Apply the 3Bs Principle™
- Keep your head, neck and back in neutral position at all times

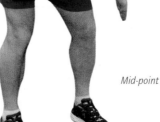

Mid-point

- Breathe out as you pull the single KB up past the body, leading with the elbow, keeping the arms close to the body at all times
- Breathe in as you lower the arm to complete one repetition
- Repeat drill with KB in opposite hand

Note: Brace your core and extend the resting arm out wide for an additional core challenge.

Double Arm Row – Neutral Grip

17. Bent Over Rows

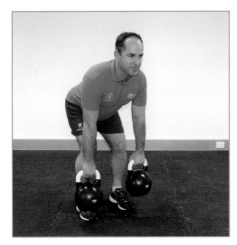
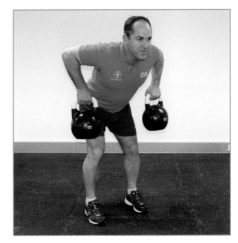

Start   *Mid-point*

Description
- Start in semi-squat position with your legs slightly bent and your back flat with your arms extended down holding KBs in both hands, knuckles forward
- Apply the 3Bs Principle™
- Raise both elbows up high in a rowing motion before lowering

Exercise variations include:

Exercise grip variations
- Knuckles facing outward – neutral grip with elbows held close to the body when lowering and raising
- Knuckles facing forward – wide grip with elbows raised high
- Reciprocal – alternate arm movements

Bench options for the above three grip variations
- Lying on your stomach on a high flat bench
- Lying on your stomach on an incline bench at slight angle

18. Bent Over Reverse Fly

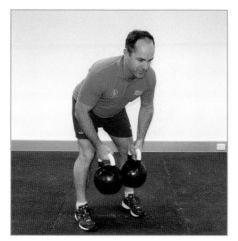

Start

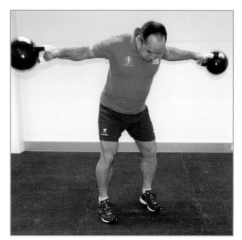

Mid-point

Description
- Stand with feet hip-width apart while gripping KBs in front of your body
- Bend at the hip and knee while leaning your torso forward until parallel with the ground and your arms are extended down in front of the body, slightly bent with knuckles facing outward
- Apply the 3Bs Principle™
- Keep your head, neck and back in neutral position at all times
- Breathe out as you raise both arms up and out wide in an arcing motion until the upper arms are parallel to the ground
- Breathe in as you lower the arms to complete one repetition

Note: This exercise can also be performed lying on your chest on a high flat bench or incline bench. During an explosive movement, the KB will line up with the arms when raised (as shown). If performing a slow, controlled movement, the KB may rotate in the hand at a 90-degree angle with the base always pointed at the ground.

19. Fitness Ball Pullovers

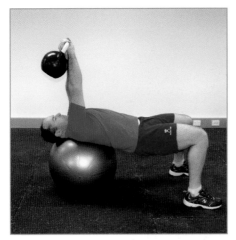

Start

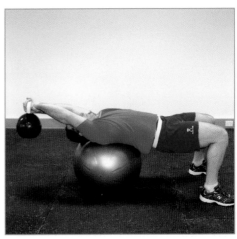

Mid-point

Description

- Lie on your back on a fitness ball along the upper back region with your arms extended vertically, slightly bent and both hands gripping the upper end of a single KB with the palms facing upward. Your knees should be bent with your feet resting on the ground
- Apply the 3Bs Principle™ – keeping hip position high and in line with the knees and shoulders
- Breathe in as you lower your arms overhead in an arcing motion while resisting any arching of the lower back until the upper arms rest beside your ears
- Breathe out as you pull the KB back up overhead to complete one repetition

Note: This exercise can also be performed lying on a flat bench or across (sideways) a flat bench, resting on your upper back with the knees bent and hips held high.

20. Single Arm Upright Row

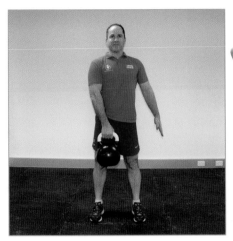

Start

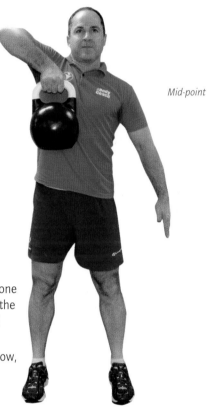

Mid-point

Description

- Stand with feet shoulder-width apart, one hand on your hip and the other gripping the KB in front of your thigh, knuckles forward
- Apply the 3Bs Principle™
- Raise your arm up, leading with the elbow, then lower
- Keep wrist straight at all times
- Repeat drill with opposite arm

Note: The progressive extension of this exercise is a high pull from the ground.

21. Upright Rows – Single KB

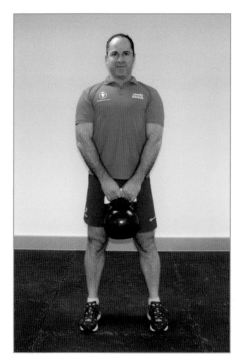 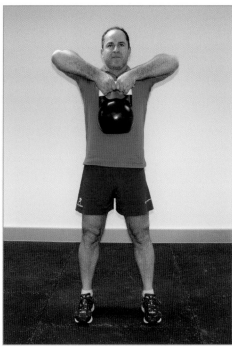

Start   Mid-point

Description
- Start in an upright standing position with feet shoulder-width apart and arms extended down in front of the thighs, gripping a single KB handle, knuckles facing forward
- Apply the 3Bs Principle™
- Leading with the elbows, breathe out as you raise the elbows up high while keeping the KB close to the body up to chest height (under the chin)
- Avoid any forward raising of the KB or bending of the wrists
- Breathe in and lower to complete one repetition

Variation
- Start in a semi-squat position with the KB lowered between your legs and simultaneously raise your body and pull the KB upward.

22. Upright Rows – Double KB

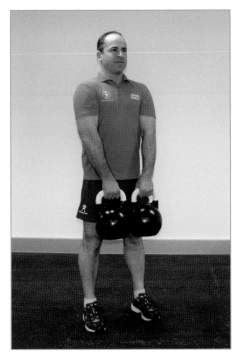 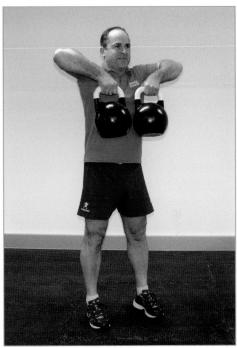

Start   *Mid-point*

Description
- Start in an upright standing position with feet shoulder-width apart and arms extended down in front of the thighs gripping KBs close together, with knuckles facing forward
- Apply the 3Bs Principle™
- Leading with the elbows, breathe out as you raise the elbows up high while keeping the KBs close to the body up to chest height (under the chin)
- Avoid any forward raising of the KBs or bending of the wrists
- Breathe in and lower to complete one repetition

Variations
- Start in a semi-squat position with both KBs lowered between the legs and simultaneously raise the body and pull the KBs upward
- This exercise can also be performed starting with a wider arm position (like holding an Olympic bar shoulder-width apart) and raising your elbows and upper arms until parallel

SHOULDERS

The deltoid (shoulder) muscle covers the shoulder and consists of three distinct segments:

1. The **anterior**, or front deltoid, allows you to raise your arm to the front.

2. The **medial**, or middle deltoid, allows you to raise your arm to the side.

3. The **posterior**, or rear deltoid, allows you to draw your arm backwards when it is perpendicular to the torso.

Different exercise movements of the shoulder target the different parts of the deltoid.

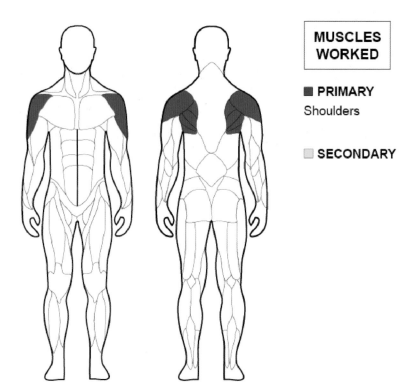

MUSCLES
WORKED

■ PRIMARY
Shoulders

☐ SECONDARY

23. Single Arm Front Raise – 1

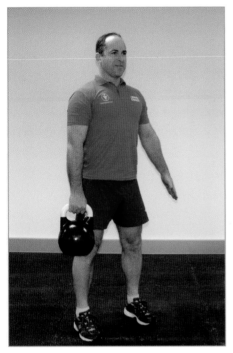

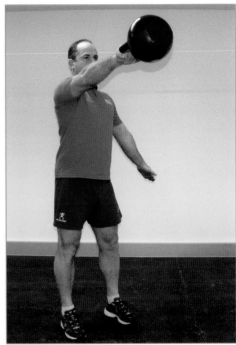

Start

Mid-point

Description
- Stand with feet shoulder-width apart, one hand on hip and the other gripping KB in front of thigh, knuckles forward
- Apply the 3Bs Principle™
- Raise one arm up in front of the body up to eye level, then lower in a controlled motion
- Repeat drill with opposite arm

Note: During an explosive movement, the KB will line up with the arm and wrist when raised (as shown). If performing a slow, controlled movement, the KB may rotate (swivel) in the hand at a 90-degree angle with the base always pointed at the ground.

24. Single Arm Front Raise – 2

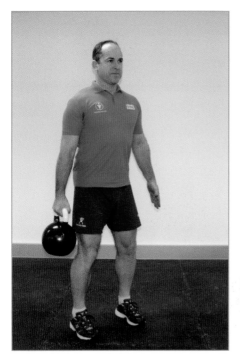
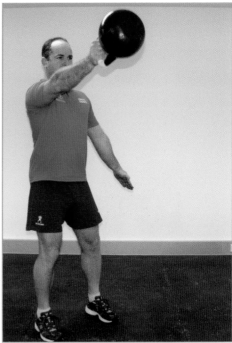

Start   *Mid-point*

Description
- Stand with feet shoulder-width apart, one hand on your hip and the other gripping the KB in front of your thigh, knuckles forward
- Apply the 3Bs Principle™
- Raise one arm up in front of the body up to eye level, then lower, allowing the KB handle to swivel in your hand
- Repeat drill with opposite arm

25. Double KB Front Raise

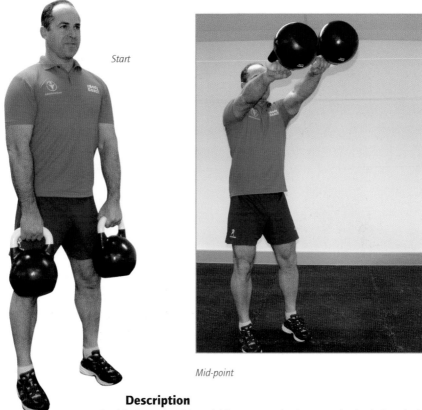

Start

Mid-point

Description
- Stand with feet shoulder-width apart, gripping KBs in both hands in front of your thighs, knuckles forward
- Apply the 3Bs Principle™
- Raise arms up in front of the body up to eye level, then lower to complete one repetition

Variations
- Knuckles face forward
- Arms resting by your side, knuckles facing outward while raising, maintaining a straight wrist at all times
- Alternate arm raise – one KB at a time

Note: During an explosive movement, the KB will line up with the arm and wrist when raised (as shown). If performing a slow, controlled movement, the KB may rotate (swivel) in the hand at a 90-degree angle with the base always pointed at the ground.

26. Single Arm Shoulder Press

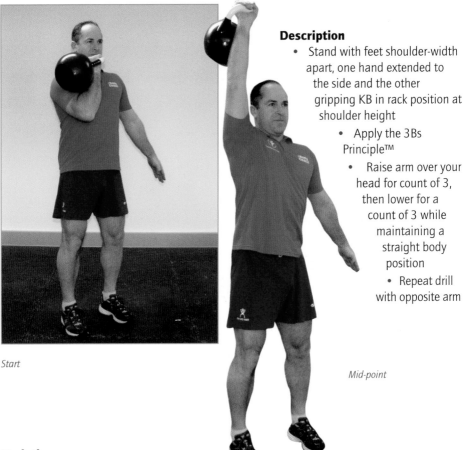

Start

Mid-point

Description

- Stand with feet shoulder-width apart, one hand extended to the side and the other gripping KB in rack position at shoulder height
- Apply the 3Bs Principle™
- Raise arm over your head for count of 3, then lower for a count of 3 while maintaining a straight body position
- Repeat drill with opposite arm

Variation

- Follow the KB with your eyes as it is raised above the head with a slight bend of the torso

27. Bottom Up Press

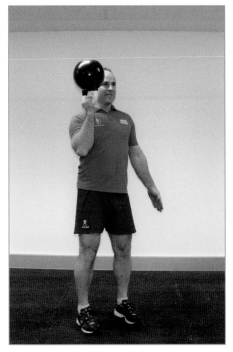
Start

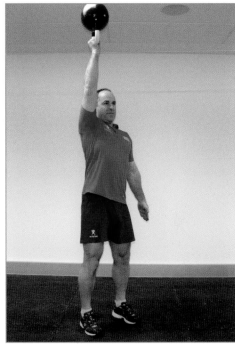
Mid-point

Description
- Stand with feet shoulder-width apart, one hand extended to the side and the other gripping the KB handle with the KB upside down (bottom up) at shoulder height
- Apply the 3Bs Principle™
- Raise your arm over your head for a count of 3, then lower it for a count of 3 while maintaining a straight body position and strong grip to avoid any movement of the KB
- Repeat drill with the opposite arm

Variation
- Follow the KB with your eyes while raised above the head while slightly bending your torso

28. Kettlebell Press

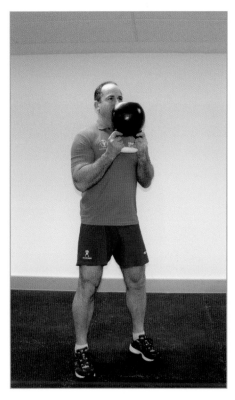

Start

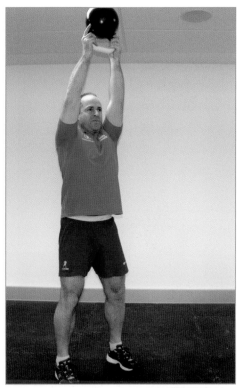

Mid-point

Description
- Stand with your feet shoulder-width apart, arms bent and both hands raised in front of your chest gripping the handles of KBs with the bottom facing up
- Apply the 3 Bs Principle™
- Raise the KBs up over your head for a count of 3, then lower them for a count of 3 while maintaining a straight body position

29. Waiter Press

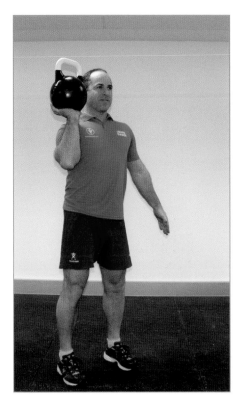

Start

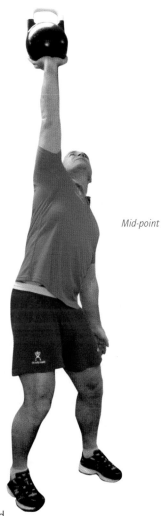

Mid-point

Description
- Stand with feet shoulder-width apart, one hand extended to the side and the other hand flat under the base of KB at shoulder height
- Apply the 3Bs Principle™
- Raise arm over your head for count of 3, then lower for a count of 3
- Follow the KB with your eyes as it is raised above the head with slight bend of torso
- Repeat drill with opposite arm

30. Fingertip Press

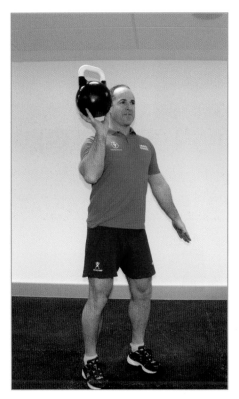

Start

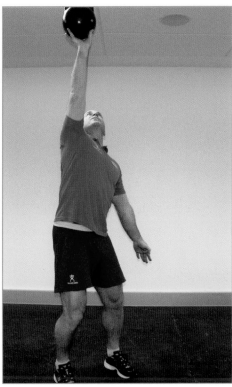

Mid-point

Description
- Stand with feet shoulder-width apart, one hand extended to the side and the other cupped with the fingers spread apart holding the base of the KB at shoulder height
- Apply the 3Bs Principle™
- Raise the arm over your head for a count of 3, then lower for a count of 3
- Follow the KB with your eyes as it is raised above your head as you slightly bend the torso
- Repeat drill with opposite arm

31. Seated KB Press

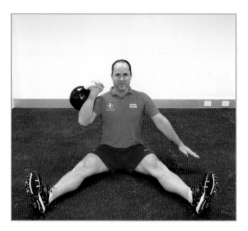

Start

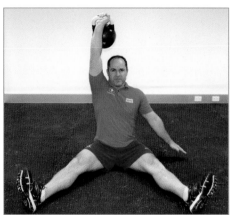

Mid-point

Description
- Sit on the ground with legs wide apart and torso erect. One arm is raised to the side gripping the KB and the other arm extended out to side
- Apply the 3Bs Principle™
- Raise the arm over your head for a count of 3, then lower for a count of 3 in a controlled manner
- Repeat drill with opposite arm

Variation
- Follow the KB with your eyes as you raise it above your head while you slightly bend your torso (as shown below). Two KBs can also be used when starting in a rack position. This requires strong abdominal bracing at all times.

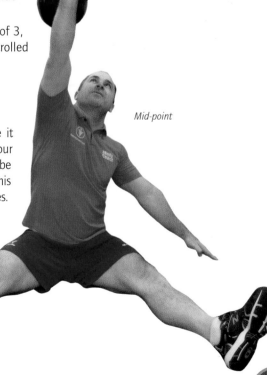

Mid-point

32. Overhead Double KB Press

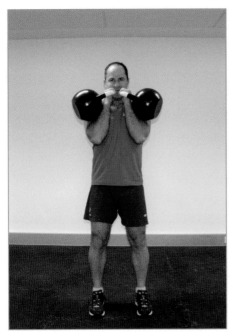

Start

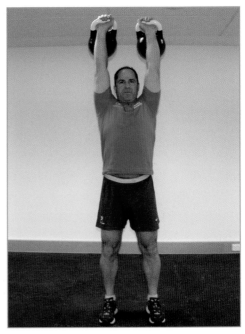

Mid-point

Description
- Stand tall with your feet shoulder-width apart, arms bent and raised, gripping two KBs in rack position at shoulder height
- Apply the 3Bs Principle™
- Breathe out as you raise both KBs over your head
- Breathe in and lower the KBs back down to shoulder height (or rack position) to complete one repetition

Variations
- Various grip positions can be applied from the starting position and when raising the KBs either straight up overhead or with an arm rotation with each exercise:
- Rack position (as shown above)
- Rack position – knuckles positioned forward
- Arms start out wide in line with the shoulders, knuckles facing backwards

Note: This exercise can also be performed sitting on a flat weight bench or fitness ball with both arms. The upward movement can also be performed simultaneously – as one arm goes up, the other lowers.

33. Overhead Double KB Alternate Press

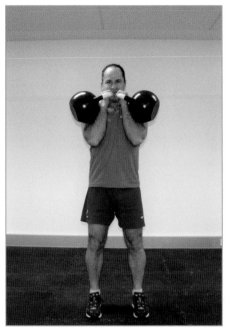

Start

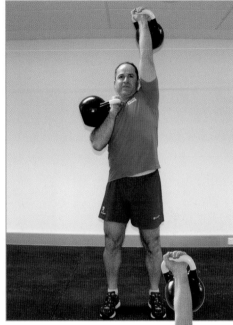

Mid-point

Description
- Stand tall with feet shoulder-width apart and arms bent and raised, gripping two KBs in rack position at shoulder height
- Apply the 3Bs Principle™
- Breath out as you raise one KB over your head
- Breathe in and lower the KB back down to shoulder height (or rack position) to complete one repetition before raising the other arm by itself

Variations
- This exercise can also be performed starting with one arm extended and the other in the rack position while moving the arms up and down simultaneously. In addition, follow the KB with your eyes as it is raised above the head with a slight bend of the torso (as shown below). This exercise can also be performed sitting on a flat weight bench or fitness ball with both arms (or alternate, single arm raises).

Mid-point

34. Lateral Raise

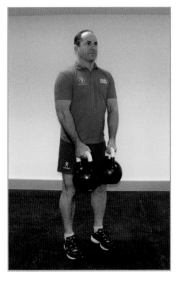

Start

Mid-point

Description
- Stand with feet together, gripping two KBs in both hands in front of your body with arms slightly bent, palms inward
- Apply the 3 Bs Principle™
- Breathe out as you raise the arms out and up to the side in a semicircular motion until your arms are parallel to the ground – keeping wrists straight and KBs in line at all times
- Avoid any forward head movement or leaning your body backwards
- Breathe in and lower the KB back down in a controlled motion to complete one repetition

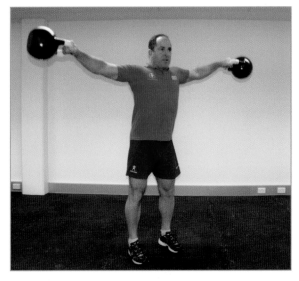

Mid-point

Note: During an explosive movement, the KB will line up with the arm and wrist when raised (as shown above). If performing a slow, controlled movement, the KB may rotate (swivel) in the hand at a 90-degree angle with the base always pointed at the ground (as shown below). Perform a single arm movement as a variation to build strength, good muscle control and to limit any forward head movement.

TRICEPS

- **Triceps** – The rear side of the upper arm.

- **Pectoralis (Chest)** – Large fan-shaped muscle that covers the front of the upper chest.

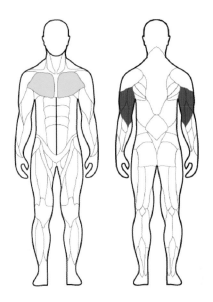

MUSCLES WORKED
■ **PRIMARY** Triceps
▩ **SECONDARY** Chest

35. Triceps Kickbacks – 1

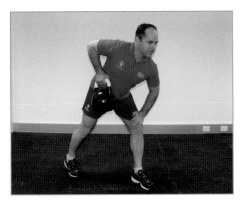
Start

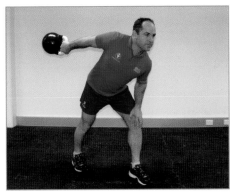
Mid-point

Description
- Stand with one leg forward and the other back
- Rest forward hand above the knee with your rear arm bent by your side at 90-degrees while holding the KB, knuckles forward
- Apply the 3Bs Principle™
- Keeping the wrist straight, extend the arm back until parallel to the ground before returning
- Repeat drill with opposite arm

Note: This exercise can also be performed with one leg kneeling on a flat bench.

36. Triceps Kickback – 2: Double KB

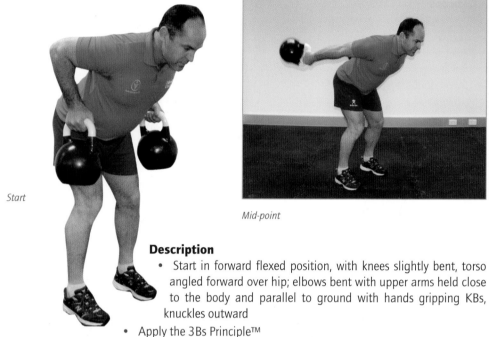

Start

Mid-point

Description

- Start in forward flexed position, with knees slightly bent, torso angled forward over hip; elbows bent with upper arms held close to the body and parallel to ground with hands gripping KBs, knuckles outward
- Apply the 3Bs Principle™
- Breathe out as you extend both hands back and up until your forearm is parallel to the ground. Be sure the wrist is kept straight at all times and the arms are close to your body
- Breathe in as you lower the KBs back down by bending the elbows to complete one repetition

Note: During an explosive movement, the KB will line up with the arm and wrist when raised (as shown above). If performing a slow, controlled movement, a lighter KB may be required to develop good muscle, forearm and wrist control before increasing weight lifted to avoid injury.

37. Triceps Extension – 1

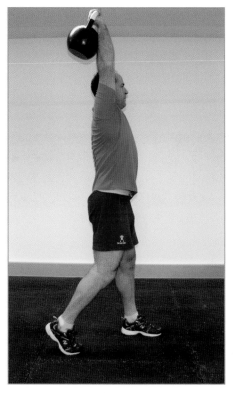

Start

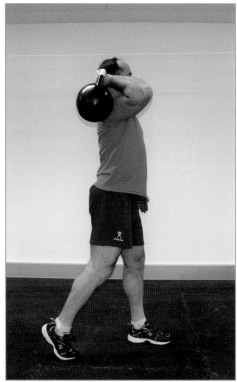

Mid-point

Description

- Stand with one leg forward and the other back resting on the toes
- Grip the KB in one hand and extend the arm up over your head with palm forward, and the other arm extended out by your side
- Apply the 3Bs Principle™
- Bend elbow and lower the KB behind your head without any change of body position before straightening your arm over your head
- Repeat the drill with the opposite arm

Variation

- Try grip variations on the handle.

38. Triceps Extension – 2

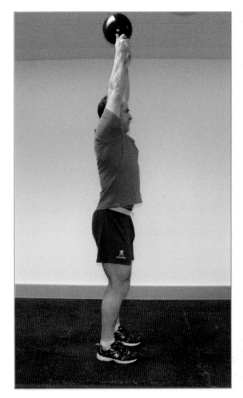

Start

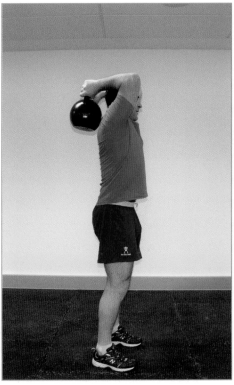

Mid-point

Description
- Start in an upright standing position with feet shoulder-width apart and both arms extended vertically while gripping the outside of the handle with both hands. The bottom of the KB should be facing upward
- Apply the 3Bs Principle™
- Breathe in as you bend the elbows and lower the KB until your forearms descend just past parallel to the ground, behind your head
- Breathe out as you raise the KB back up to the vertical starting position to complete one repetition with wrists straight
- Ensure strong abdominal bracing at all times to avoid lower back arching – adjust accordingly

Note: This exercise can also be performed kneeling, seated on a flat weight bench or fitness ball or standing in a lunge position.

39. Triceps Extension – 3: Double KB

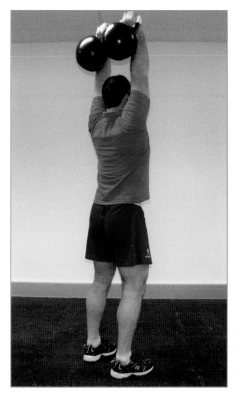
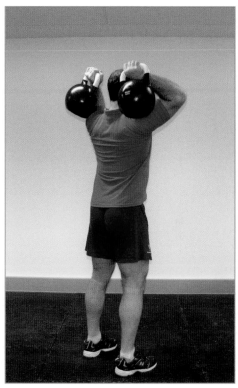

Start   *Mid-point*

Description

- Start in an upright standing position with feet shoulder-width apart and both arms extended vertically, gripping KBs with knuckles facing backwards
- Apply the 3 Bs Principle™
- Breathe in as you bend the elbows and lower both arms until the forearms descend just past parallel to the ground, behind your head
- Breathe out as you raise the KBs back up to the vertical starting position to complete one repetition
- Ensure strong abdominal bracing at all times to avoid lower back arching – adjust accordingly

Note: This exercise can also be performed seated on a flat weight bench or fitness ball or standing in a forward lunge position.

40. Triceps French Press – 1: Single KB

Description
- Lie on your back on the ground with knees bent
- Extend one arm directly above your shoulder, gripping KB and the other arm down by your side
- Apply the 3Bs Principle™

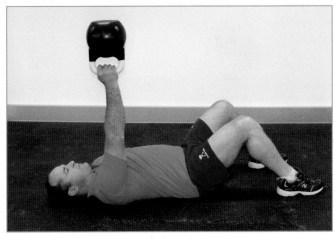

Start

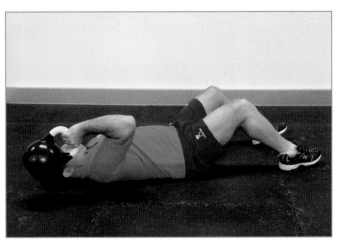

Mid-point

- Keeping the wrist straight, extend the arm back until it is parallel to the ground before returning. Be sure the wrist remains straight at all times
- Repeat drill with the opposite arm

Variation
- Double KB triceps French press

41. Triceps French Press – 2: Double KB

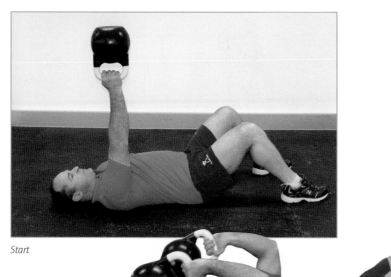

Start

Mid-point

Description

- Lie on your back on the ground with knees bent
- Extend both arms directly above your shoulder gripping a KB in each hand while maintaining a straight wrist and strong grip with the bottom of the KB facing upward
- Apply the 3Bs Principle™
- Keeping the wrist straight, extend both arms back until parallel to the ground before returning. Be sure the wrists remain straight at all times

Variation

- Apply triceps extension – 3: Double KB in a lying position

BICEPS

- **Biceps –** The front side of the upper arm, which bends and supinates the elbow

- **Forearms –** Collective muscle between the elbow and wrist that bends the elbow, which pronates and supinates the elbow depending on the starting position

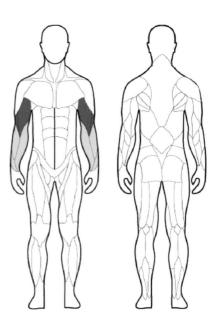

MUSCLES WORKED

■ **PRIMARY**
Biceps

☐ **SECONDAR**
Forearms

42. Single KB Biceps Curl

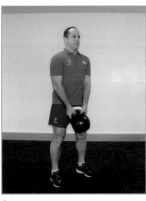

Start

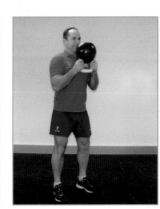

Mid-point

Description
- Stand tall with feet shoulder-width apart and both arms extended down, gripping the outside of the KB handle in front of your body
- Apply the 3Bs Principle™

- Breathe out as you simultaneously bend your elbows and curl the KB up to shoulder height. Keep your wrists straight and upper arms held close to the body
- Breathe in as you lower the KB down to your thigh to complete one repetition

43. Hammer Curl

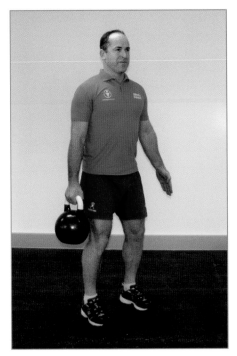

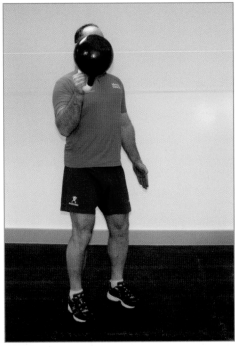

Start   *Mid-point*

Description
- Stand tall with feet shoulder-width apart and one arm extended down, gripping the KB by your side with the knuckles facing out and the other arm out by your side
- Apply the 3Bs Principle™
- Breathe out as you simultaneously bend your elbow and curl the KB up to shoulder height. Keep your wrists straight, knuckles out and upper arm held close by your side
- Breathe in as you lower the KB in a controlled motion down by your thigh to complete one repetition
- Repeat with opposite arm

Variations
- Double KB alternate arm hammer curls
- Double KB hammer curls
- Use a lunge stance

44. Open Curls

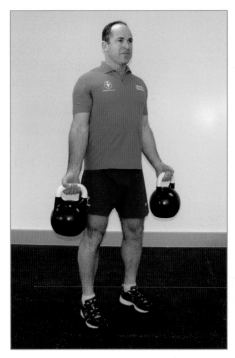

Start

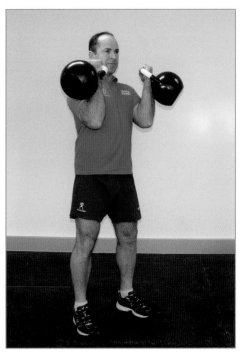

Mid-point

Description
- Stand tall with feet shoulder-width apart and arms extended down resting KBs by your side with palms facing forward and upper arms held in close to your body
- Apply the 3Bs Principle™
- Breathe out as you simultaneously bend your elbows and curl both KBs up to shoulder height. Keep your wrists straight at all times while allowing the KBs to rotate through your hands
- Breathe in as you lower the KBs down outside of your thighs to complete one repetition

Variations
- Single arm KB open curls
- Double KB alternate arm open curls
- Use a lunge stance

45. Rotation Curls

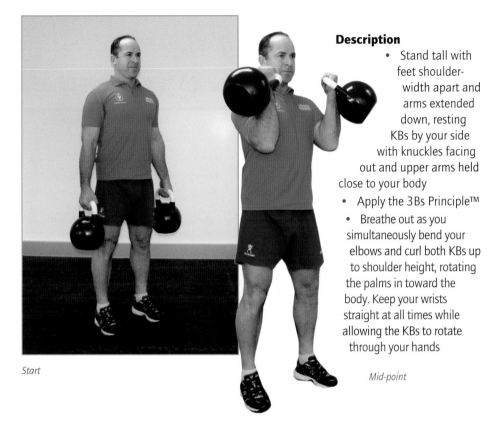

Start

Mid-point

Description
- Stand tall with feet shoulder-width apart and arms extended down, resting KBs by your side with knuckles facing out and upper arms held close to your body
- Apply the 3Bs Principle™
- Breathe out as you simultaneously bend your elbows and curl both KBs up to shoulder height, rotating the palms in toward the body. Keep your wrists straight at all times while allowing the KBs to rotate through your hands

- Breathe in as you lower and rotate your forearms and KBs back down outside of your thighs with knuckles facing outward to complete one repetition

Note: This exercise can also be performed seated or in a standing lunge stance position, using a single arm or both arms simultaneously.

Variations
- Single arm KB rotation curl
- Double KB alternate arm rotation curls
- Use a lunge stance
- Seated

LEGS

Teaching Points
- Apply the 3Bs Principle™ with each exercise
- Keep chest erect and aim to make movement flow efficiently
- Keep knees over the midline of the toes
- Ensure good ankle, knee, hip and body alignment is maintained when lowering and raising the body
- Maintain a strong pelvic position parallel to the ground at all times without allowing the pelvis to tilt or lower
- Maintain deep breathing pattern at all times
- Breathe out when rising
- Breathe in when lowering
- Stop exercise if any lower back or knee tension or pain arises
- Always have a coach or personal trainer assist in demonstrating, teaching and spotting each exercise

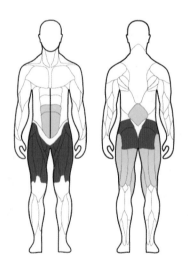

MUSCLES WORKED

■ **PRIMARY**
Quadriceps
Glutes

▢ **SECONDARY**
Hamstrings
Abdominals
Lower Back

This section combines the muscles of the leg and hip regions:
- **Quadriceps** – This is the large group of muscles on the front of the upper leg, referred to as the thighs. These muscles start at the hip joint and end at the knee joint. Their primary function is to flex the hip and extend the knee, which is very important in walking, running, jumping, climbing and pedalling a bike.
- **Hamstrings** – This is the group of muscles on the backside of the leg, running from the hip joint to the knee joint. Their primary function is to facilitate the flexing of the legs and medial and lateral rotation. They are important for walking, running and jumping.
- **Gluteal Region** – Often referred to as the buttocks region, the primary function is hip extension in unison with the hip stabilizers. This is important in all lower-body movements.
- **Lower Back** – There are several muscles in the lower back (lumbar region) that assist with rotation, flexibility and strength. This is generally the area of the torso between the diaphragm and the sacrum on the back side of the body from which muscle and fascia attach.

Deadlifts

46. Wheelbarrow Deadlift

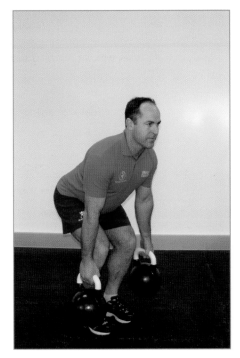

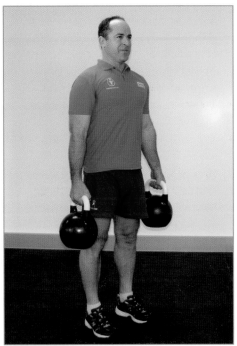

Start   *Mid-point*

Description
- Start in a squat position with feet shoulder-width apart, back flat and arms extended down outside the legs, gripping KBs. They should be held around ankle height with knuckles facing out, as if you were holding wheelbarrow handles (though in a lower starting position)
- The range of motion through the hip and lower back region in a squat position will depend on one's flexibility, coordination and muscle control
- Apply the 3Bs Principle™
- Driving through the legs, push the body up until your legs are straight
- Ensure the KBs remain close to your legs as you rise
- Once standing, pause briefly, then reverse the movement back down to the starting position to complete one repetition

47. Romanian Deadlift

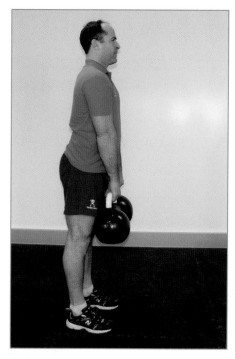

Start

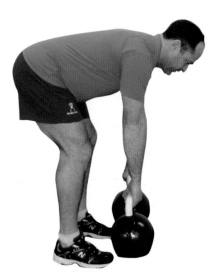

Mid-point

Description
- Start in an upright standing position, arms extended down gripping a KB with each hand. Rest the KBs on your thighs with knuckles facing forward
- Applying the 3Bs Principle™, brace the core-abdominal muscles
- Keeping your back flat, bend forward at the hips while slightly bending at the knees. Lower the body until the torso is parallel to the ground
- Ensure your head and neck remain aligned (neutral) with your body when leaning forward
- Once lowered, pause briefly, then reverse the movement back up ensuring the abdominals remain braced as you return to the upright starting position to complete one repetition

Variation
- A more advanced version of this exercise involves keeping your legs straight at all times

48. Sumo Deadlift

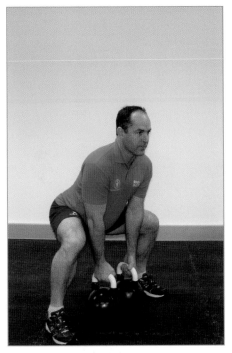 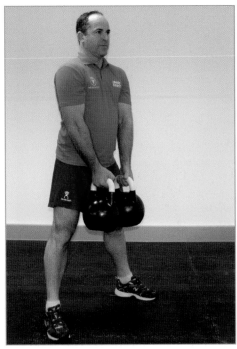

Start   Mid-point

Description
- Start with two KBs on the ground in front of your body with handles aligned
- Widen your feet on either side of the KBs and bend at the ankles, knees and hips in a wide sumo squat position with arms straight and extended down, gripping a KB in each hand The palms should face inward
- Apply the 3Bs Principle™
- Driving through the legs, push your body up until standing tall with the arms remaining straight at all times, close to the body
- Once standing, pause briefly, then reverse the movement back down to the starting position to complete one repetition

Variation
- Single KB sumo deadlift

49. Single Leg Dead-lift – 1

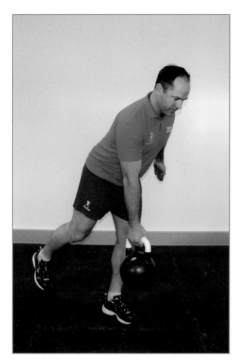 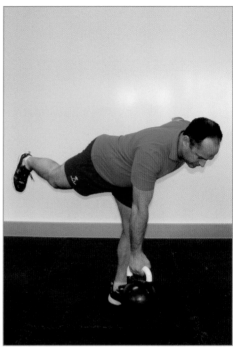

Start   *Mid-point*

Description
- Stand on one leg with opposite arm extended down, holding a KB, knuckles outward
- Extend the opposite arm out to your side for balance and raise the rear leg slightly off the ground behind your body
- Apply the 3Bs Principle™
- Keeping your back flat and hips square, breathe in as you lower forward until your back is almost parallel to ground
- Pause briefly before breathing out and rising back up to complete one repetition
- Ensure good ankle, knee, hip and body alignment is maintained when lowering and raising the torso and rear leg
- Repeat drill on the opposite side

Variation
- Hold a KB in both hands in front of the body and lower and rise

50. Single Leg Dead-lift – 2: Double KB

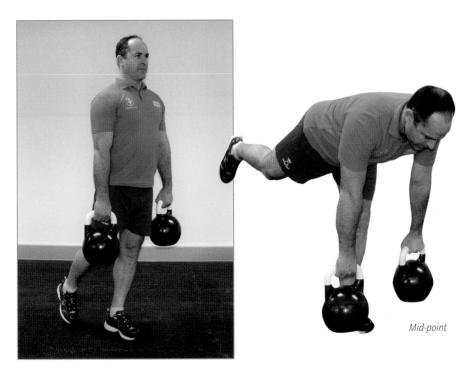

Mid-point

Start

Description

- Gripping KBs in each hand by your side, with knuckles facing out, balance on the left leg with the right leg raised slightly off ground behind the body
- Apply the 3Bs Principle™
- Keeping your back flat and legs straight, bend forward at the hips, lowering the body until the torso is parallel to the ground
- To increase the challenge, also raise the rear leg until parallel while ensuring the hips remain square
- Ensure your head and neck remain neutral to your body while the arms are extended down
- Once lowered, pause briefly, then reverse the movement back up making sure the hips remain square and the abdominals braced as you move back up to the starting position to complete one repetition
- Ensure good ankle, knee, hip and body alignment is maintained when lowering and raising the torso and rear leg
- Repeat movement balancing on right leg

Lunges

51. Stationary Lunge

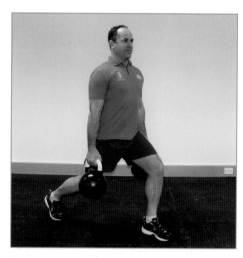

Start

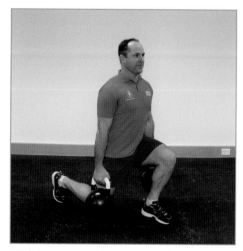

Mid-point

Description

- Stand tall in forward lunge position with one leg forward and the other back behind the body resting on the toes. The arms should extend down either side of the body, gripping KBs
- Apply the 3Bs Principle™
- Tilt the pelvis back, brace the abdominals and square the hips to ensure correct torso positioning during movement and to avoid any arching of the lower back region
- Breathe in as you lower the rear knee toward the ground and as the front thigh becomes parallel to the ground with your knees over your toes
- Breathe out and rise up to complete one repetition
- Repeat drill with opposite leg forward

Note: See multiple exercise variations on the following pages.

52. Stationary Lunge Variations – Starting Positions

Arm and hand positioning plays a major role in determining the challenge placed on the legs, posture and core region in lunge exercises. The following illustrates variations of a stationary lunge starting position. See Stationary Lunge Exercise description on the previous page. Repeat exercise with opposite leg forward. For additional variation of these exercises, the rear leg may also be placed on a flat weight bench to increase the intensity.

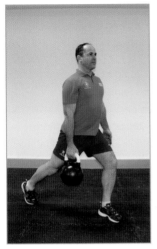

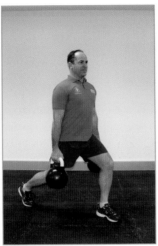

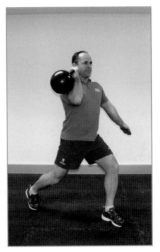

A. One arm is extended down by side gripping KB, knuckles facing out; opposite arm is held out to the side for balance

B. Both arms are extended down by the sides, gripping KBs, knuckles facing out (as previously prescribed)

C. One hand holds the KB in rack position; the opposite arm is extended out to the side for balance

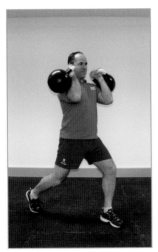

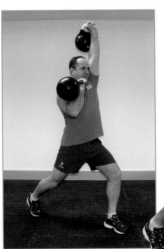

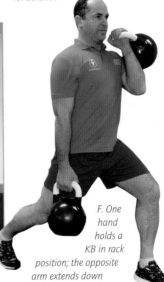

D. Both hands are holding KBs in rack position. Arm movements made from this position may be single or double

E. One hand holds a KB in rack position; opposite arm extended over the head holding the KB

F. One hand holds a KB in rack position; the opposite arm extends down holding the KB by the side, knuckles facing outwards

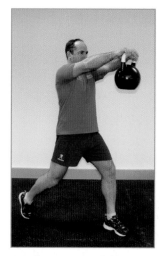

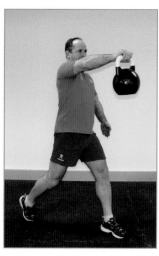

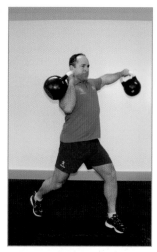

G. Both arms are extended forward holding one KB

H. Extend the opposite arm forward, parallel to ground while holding the KB with the other arm out to the side for balance

I. One hand holds the KB in rack position; the opposite arm is extended laterally to the side of the body while gripping the KB, knuckles facing up

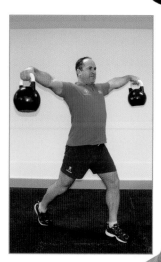

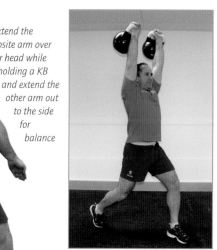

K. Extend the opposite arm over your head while holding a KB and extend the other arm out to the side for balance

J. Both arms are extended laterally to the sides of the body while gripping the KB, knuckles facing up

L. Both arms are extended over your head while gripping KBs

As with any exercise, stop the exercise immediately or readjust the body constantly using the 3Bs Principle™ once the core bracing is lost, or poor posture, poor alignment or fatigue sets in. Be sure to value quality of movement over quantity. Reduce the KB weight being used to ensure good posture at all times before increasing.

53. Alternate Leg Lunge

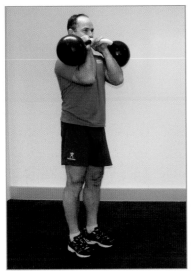

Start

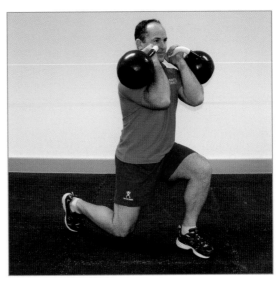

Mid-point

Description
- Stand tall with your feet close together and your hands gripping KBs in rack position in front of your body
- Apply the 3Bs Principle™
- Breathe in as you step forward with one leg into a lunge position until the front thigh is parallel to the ground, knee over toes, and the rear knee is close to the ground
- Breathe out as you push back up off the front leg to the upright starting position to complete one repetition
- Repeat drill with the opposite leg lunging forward

Variations
- Walking lunge – continuously walk forward
- Backwards lunge
- Diagonal lunge
- Side lunge
- Step-ups – onto bench
- Lateral step-overs – across bench
- Lunge press – forward lunge with a single arm press overhead from rack position

Note: See stationary lunge variations for additional arm starting positions for a greater challenge to the legs and core region.

Squats

Squat Patterning

Squat exercises are the foundation for a wide variety of sporting skills, from exploding out of the blocks in the 100m dash to jumping, landing and stepping. The squat itself is a highly effective measure of muscular balance, coordination and flexibility due to the requirement of depth, control and body positioning.

The squat movement generally ranges from a half-squat (90-degree leg angle) to a full or deep squat position, as required in Olympic lifting. Working between these ranges will depend on one's coordination, strength, control and flexibility. These elements, along with a person's age and bio-mechanical efficiency, need to be taken into consideration with the actual squat depth performed and will need to be assessed and approved by a physical therapist or qualified strength and conditioning coach or personal trainer. These considerations are designed to protect one's lower back, knees and ankles from injury.

Once a good squat pattern is obtained through body weight movements and stretching (or stability drills), the weight of the kettlebells used can be increased for strength improvements. Always apply the 3Bs Principle™ to ensure correct body posture, breathing and movement patterns in squat exercises.

Good Body Alignment

Ultimately, one's goal in squatting is to effectively activate the glutes, hamstrings and thigh muscles. This is achieved through the initial activation of the hips and knees by pushing the glutes back and keeping the back flat while the knees remain over the toes from both the side and front perspectives.

Good Postural Alignment
The most common mistakes to avoid in squatting are:
* **Bending primarily at the ankles first** – This limits the range of motion at this joint and leads to the heels rising off the ground or knees rolling inward to accommodate any further squatting movement to follow. This may also lead to a more upright body position as opposed to shoulder over knee. For this reason, participants with flat feet, weak knees or poor squat initiation at the ankles need to concentrate on keeping their weight distributed across the foot (establishing a foot arch)

Good Squat Alignment

Side Position	Front Position
• Ear over shoulder	• Knees aligned over toes
• Shoulder over knee	• Weight across foot print
• Knee over toes	
• Feet flat on ground	

and centred; with the initial activation, knees should be aligned over the toes at the hips and knees simultaneously (as shown in the photo above)

Note: Ankle and knee alignment will vary at times due to ones ankle dorsi-flexion and hamstrings length

- **Bending too far forward at the hips** – This leads to overloading the lower back region

The squat itself is a key functional movement. In order to improve the mistakes described above and others, you can practice the supported squat exercise to learn good technique, as outlined in the proceeding pages.

Supported Squat

Description
- To assist with squat development, stand next to a pole (or door frame)
- Stand with your feet shoulder-width apart, holding the pole with both hands
- Apply the 3Bs Principle™ and establish good foot arch and knee alignment by bringing awareness to the movement that follows
- Using your hands as a support guide only, simultaneously bend at the hips and knees and lower your body by pushing the glutes back while your shoulders remain over your knees, and the knees are over the toes. Trail your hands down the pole with your body for initial support.
- Keep head close to the pole when lowering and focus on adjusting your body to maintain a good body position – ear over shoulder, over knee, over toes

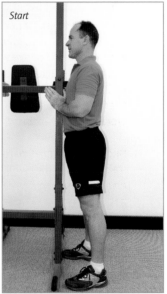

Start

Note:
- Using a pole for support enables you to improve the technical aspect of squatting by forcing you to push back through your glutes while limiting your ability to bend too far forward at the hip and shoulders. Instead, you will establish good body alignment
- This is a great warm-up drill prior to any exercise, especially free weight training. Once learned, you may move away from the pole and repeat the squat movement using your body weight only, and with the arms extended forward, parallel to ground.
- Master this drill before adding any weight to the squat movement
- Use regular stretching and massage to maintain good muscle pliability for all exercises
- Initially lower down into a short range of motion until your strength, flexibility or stability improves. Gradually lower deeper as your muscles and joints allow, under the guidance of a physical therapist or qualified coach

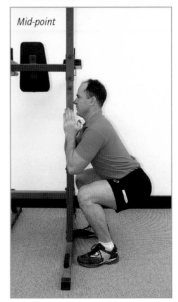

Mid-point

Squat Depth

In most exercises, squat depth is when the thighs have lowered until parallel to the ground or in half-squat position, which ensures good posture is maintained. On the other hand, completing a full squat will often depend on one's body type, flexibility, stability and sporting needs. For instance, an Olympic lifter, lifting tremendous loads, requires incredible flexibility and joint stability for his sport and thus needs a full squat training focus. A swimmer, on the other hand, may also have good flexibility or hypermobility of a joint or series of joints, but this sport doesn't require lifting tremendous loads. Hence the focus is on obtaining joint stability by performing squat exercises through a full range with good posture using lighter KBs and maintaining good body awareness. Other athletes with a rugby background, for instance, may be lacking flexibility in certain joints throughout the body, thus limiting a full range of squat motion. Either way, one must always be aware that in any training environment, athletes will vary in their range of squat motion. Therefore, it is good practice to assess and constant monitor each athlete to reduce and avoid any overuse, stress or injury while furthering athlete development.

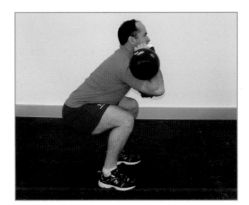

Half Squat

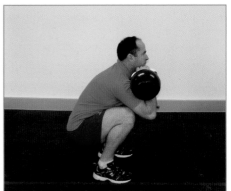

Full Squat

Note: In the full squat with KBs (demonstrated above) note that my limited ankle dorsi-flexion causes rounding of the back in order to maintain my centre of gravity as I lower deep into a squat. After 25 years of playing rugby my ankle dorsi-flexion is generally set. As one reaches an age where our body has generally established its range of motion limitations, working beyond this without appropriate guidance or understanding, as well as appropriate warming up, cooling down, stretching and massage may lead to long-term injury. In this instance, my end range of motion for a full squat will be associated to my ability to maintain a flat back and strong position. For some, it may be limited ankle dorsi-flexion and for others limited hamstrings length or poor movement mechanics. Anyone in this category must be cautious in their training to avoid overtraining or overloading, which leads to lower back stress. This is where the confusion often lies in whether one should do a half or full squat. Just remember, everyone has a different range of motion capabilities. So, for squats, always ensure you work with a qualified strength and conditioning coach to see what range is right for you based on your ankle, hamstrings and hip flexibility.

54. Bench Squat

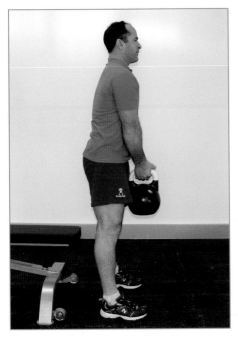
Start

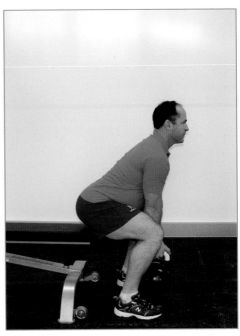
Mid-point

Description
- Start in an upright standing position in front of a weight bench, with your feet shoulder-width apart and arms extended, gripping the KB between your legs
- Apply the 3Bs Principle™ while aligning your feet and knees to create a natural foot arch and good alignment
- Breathing in, slowly squat down while simultaneously bending at the hip, knees and ankles while maintaining a flat back position
- Lower your body until your glutes touch the bench, the thighs are almost parallel to the ground, and the arms remain straight
- The bench is just a reminder of your end point when lowering, so as soon as you touch it, rise straight up again. Avoid any sitting or unloading
- Breathe out as you raise your body up, using your legs to return to the starting position to complete one repetition
- Ensure your heels remain on the floor and your knees are aligned over the toes at all times

Variation
- Hold double kettlebells by your sides with a closer foot stance.

Note: One's back position will often be determined by many factors including, but not limited to: ankle dorsi-flexion range, hamstrings length, hip mobility, balance, strength and co-ordination

55. Single Leg Bench Squat

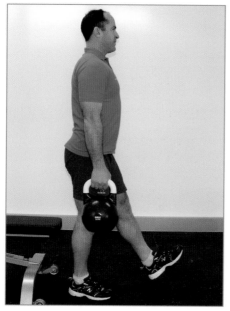

Start

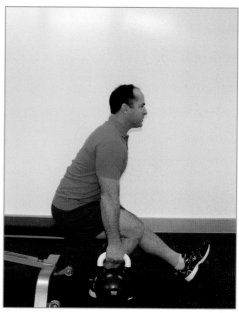

Mid-point

Description

- Start in an upright, standing position in front of a weight bench, with arms extended down by your sides, gripping KBs. One foot is raised slightly off the ground in front of the body
- Apply the 3Bs Principle™ while aligning feet and knees for natural foot arch and good alignment
- Breathing in, slowly squat down by simultaneously bending at the hip, knees and ankles while maintaining a flat back and ensuring the hips remain square and knees are aligned over the toes
- Lower your body down until your glutes touch the bench, thighs almost parallel to the ground, and the arms remain straight
- The bench is just a reminder of your end point when lowering, so as soon as you touch it, rise straight up again. Avoid any sitting or unloading
- Breathe out as you raise your body up using your legs to return to the starting position and complete one repetition
- Repeat single leg bench squat on opposite leg

Variation

- Hand position variations (see stationary lunge variations)

Note: One's back position will often be determined by many factors including, but not limited to: ankle dorsi-flexion range, hamstrings length, hip mobility, balance, strength and co-ordination

56. Front Squat – Single Rack Position

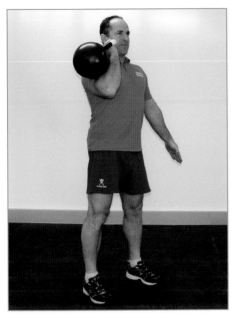

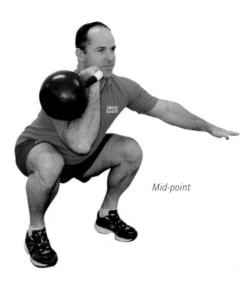

Mid-point

Start

Description
- Stand with your feet shoulder-width apart, one arm extended out to the side for balance and the other gripping a KB at shoulder height in rack position
- Apply the 3Bs Principle™
- Breathing in, slowly squat down until the thighs parallel to the ground by simultaneously bending at the hips, knees and ankles while maintaining a flat back
- Breathe out as you raise your body up using your legs to return to the starting position and complete one repetition. Squeeze your glutes as you rise
- Ensure your heels remain on the floor and the knees are aligned over the toes at all times.
- Repeat the drill with a KB in the opposite hand

Variations
- Double KB rack position
- Deep squat for more advanced athletes with good strength, control and flexibility

57. Front Squat – Double KB Rack Position

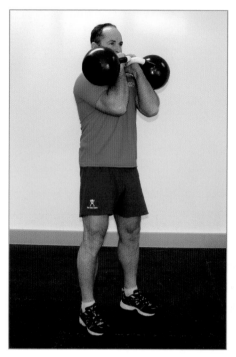

Start

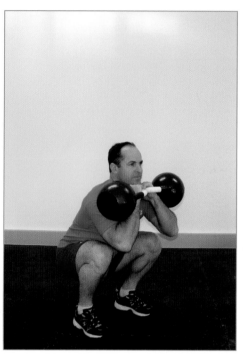

Lowered

Description
- Stand with your feet shoulder-width apart, with two KBs resting in the rack position in front of your body
- Apply the 3Bs Principle™
- Breathing in, slowly squat down until the thighs parallel to the ground by simultaneously bending at the hips, knees and ankles while maintaining a flat back
- Breathe out as you raise your body up using your legs to return to the starting position and complete one repetition. Squeeze your glutes as you rise
- Ensure your heels remain on the floor and the knees are aligned over the toes at all times

Variation
- Deep squat for more advanced athletes with good strength, control and flexibility

58. Overhead Squat

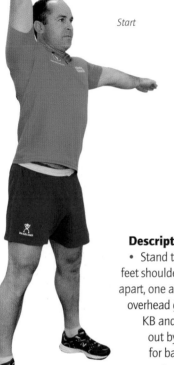

Start

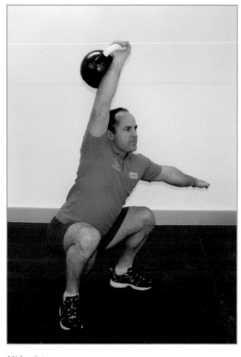

Description
• Stand tall with your feet shoulder-width apart, one arm extended overhead gripping a KB and the other out by your side for balance

Mid-point

• Apply the 3Bs Principle™ while aligning your feet and knees to obtain a natural foot arch and good alignment
• Breathing in, slowly squat down to a half-squat or full-squat position by simultaneously bending at the hips, knees and ankles while maintaining a flat back position and keeping the KB extended over your head
• Ensure the KB is held directly over your shoulder for good stability at all times
• Breathe out as you raise your body up, using your legs, to the starting position to complete one repetition. Squeeze your glutes as you rise
• Look forward or above the horizon for better movement control with your weight in front of your body
• Good shoulder flexibility and strength is required for muscle control of the KBs. Hence, always start with a light KB and master the exercise before progressing

Note: This is an advanced exercise, so ensure good flexibility and muscle control of the upper back and shoulders, as well as the hips and legs.

59. Squat Exercise – Variations

In addition to the previous exercises, variations of the squat exercise using KBs revolve around the position of the KB(s) itself and the demand it places on the core region, glutes and legs due to the changes of one's center of gravity, and the demand placed on the core region and your personal range of motion. The following exercises outline the various challenges of using different KB holding positions in squat exercises.

A. Wide Squat
legs wide, arms
extended down
holding single KB

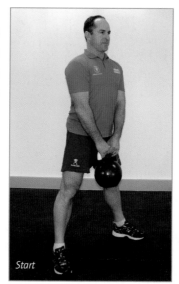

Start

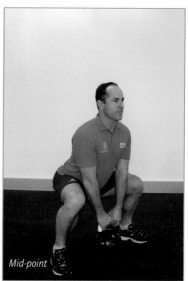

Mid-point

B. Close Grip Squat
arms bent with KB
held close to body

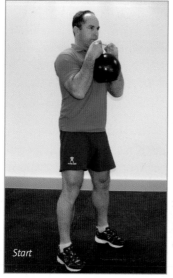

Start

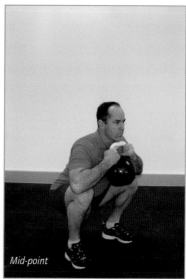

Mid-point

C. Deck Squat
arms extended
forward holding KB

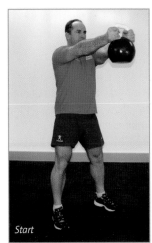
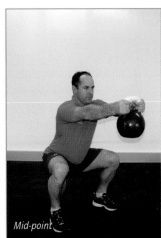

Start *Mid-point*

D. Back Squat
KBs resting on back
side of the shoulders

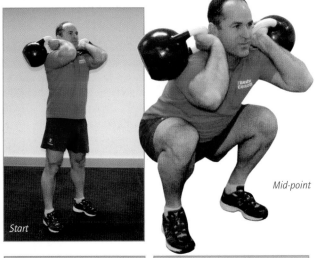

Start *Mid-point*

E. Single Leg Squat
front hold

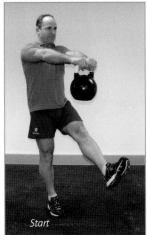
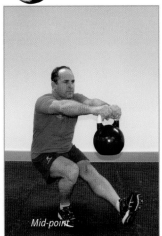

Start *Mid-point*

CALVES

- **Calves** – The group of muscles on the back of the leg running from the backside of the knee to the Achilles tendon, which bends the knee and points the toes (plantar flexion), helps us in walking, running, pedaling a bike and jumping.
- **Soleus** – The flat muscle underneath the calf muscle, which controls the ankle joint and points the toes.

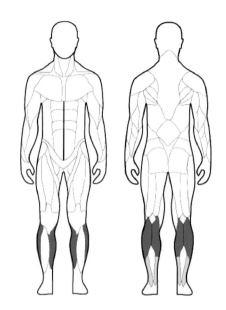

MUSCLES WORKED

■ **PRIMARY**
Calves

□ **SECONDARY**
Soleus

60. Standing Calf Raise

Description
- Stand tall with your feet hip-width apart and arms extended down the side of your body, gripping KBs
- Apply the 3Bs Principle™
- Breathing out, simultaneously rise up onto the balls of both feet, raising your heels as high as possible without losing balance
- Pause briefly at the top of movement before breathing in as you slowly lower your heels back down to the ground to complete one repetition

Variation
- This exercise can also be performed with the balls of both feet resting over the edge of a step while raising and lowering. Hold a weighted KB in one hand and grip something for support with the other hand.

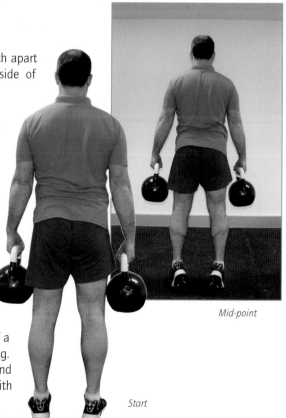

Mid-point

Start

61. Balance Calf-Raise

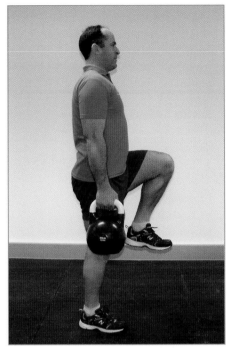
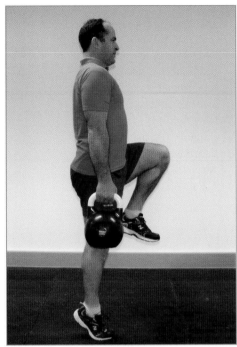

Start

Mid-point

Description
- Stand tall with your feet hip-width apart and arms extended down the side of your body, gripping KBs
- Raise one knee until it is parallel with the ground and apply the 3Bs Principle™
- Breathing out, rise up onto the ball of the foot, raising your heel as high as possible without losing balance
- Pause briefly at the top of movement before breathing in as you slowly lower your heel back down to the ground to complete one repetition
- Repeat with opposite leg

Note: A single KB may be used to allow support of the opposite hand until you have mastered the exercise or can add weight. Variations of the hand positions can also challenge your core while strengthening the calf muscles.

ABS & CORE

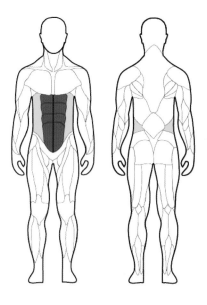

MUSCLES WORKED

■ **PRIMARY**
Abdominals

□ **SECONDARY**
Obliques

The abdominal and lower back muscles combine to form the core region of the body. The core region helps stabilize the body for more efficient and effective movement patterns to occur between the upper and lower body.

Rectus Abdominis
• Flex the trunk

Obliques
• Rotate, flex, side bend torso. Support viscera and assist exhalation

Iliopsoas
• Flexes hip

Lower Back
• Extend the spine backwards, some side bend and spinal rotation

62. KB Sit Ups

Description
• Lie on your back with one arm extended above shoulder, gripping a KB
• Bend the same leg as your raised arm and extend the other leg down with the opposite arm
• Raise the shoulder off the ground and raise the KB straight up using the abdominal muscles, then lower
• Continue looking up at the KB throughout the exercise
• Repeat on the opposite side

Variations
• Keep your free arm on your chest for additional rotation of the torso across the midline of the body.
• Cross-crunch: Raise the opposite leg in the air and reach up and across to your raised foot with the KB, then lower to strengthen the rectus abdominis and oblique muscles.

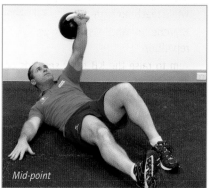

Start

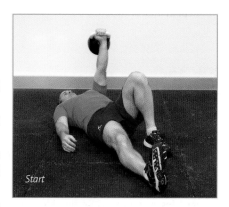

Mid-point

63. KB Sit Up Rotation

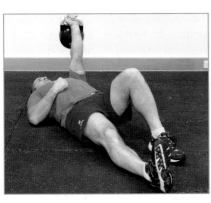

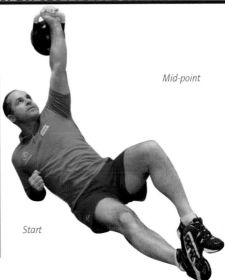

Mid-point

Start

Description

- Lie on your back with one arm extended above your shoulder, gripping a KB
- Bend the same leg as the raised arm and rest opposite elbow beside the body
- Using the abdominal muscles and opposite elbow for leverage, raise the shoulder off the ground to lift the KB straight up, then lower
- Continue looking up at the KB throughout the exercise
- Repeat on the opposite side

64. Abdominal Toe Touch

Description

- Lie on the ground with both legs raised and slightly bent
- Clasp a KB with both hands and raise the arms
- Apply the 3Bs Principle™
- While breathing out, contract the abdominal muscles and raise your shoulders off the ground while reaching high with the KB toward your feet
- Breathe in and slowly lower to complete one repetition
- Aim to raise the KB for 2 seconds or more and lower for 2 seconds or more to complete one repetition. This develops good muscle contraction

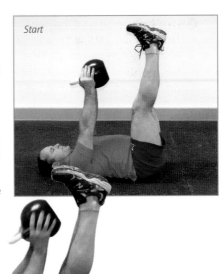

Start

Mid-point

65. Overhead Toe Touch

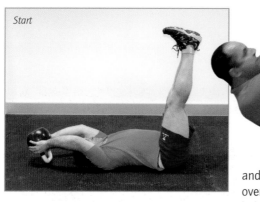

Start

Mid-point

Description
- Lie on your back with your legs raised from the hip at 90 degrees and slightly bent. Arms are extended overhead on the ground, gripping a single KB in both hands around its belly
- Apply the 3Bs Principle™
- While breathing out, simultaneously raise the KB, arms and shoulders off the ground by contracting the abdominal region. The KB should be reaching toward your raised feet
- Breathe in and slowly lower to complete one repetition
- Aim to raise the KB for 2 seconds or more and lower for 2 seconds or more to complete one repetition. This develops good muscle contraction

66. Abdominal Clams

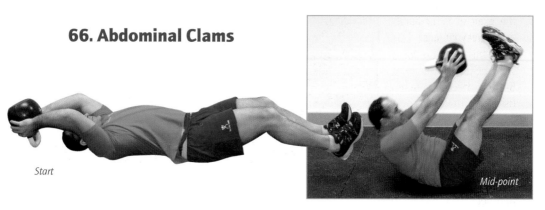

Start

Mid-point

Description
- Lie on the ground with your arms and legs extended. With both hands over your head, clasp a KB around its belly
- Apply the 3Bs Principle™
- While breathing out, contract your abdominal muscles and raise the shoulders and legs simultaneously off the ground. Reaching high with the KB toward your feet
- Breathe in and slowly lower to complete one repetition

67. Body Dish

Description

- Lie on the ground with your arms and legs extended. With both hands over your head, clasp a KB around its belly. Keep your arms pressed against your ears
- Apply the 3Bs Principle™
- Simultaneously raise your arms and legs into a body dish (banana shape) position and hold
- Keep the body long and extended to ensure the abdominals are activated. The lower back must remain in contact with the floor at all times. The toe of the raised leg is pointed. If you cannot hold these positions, stop the exercise immediately and lower your legs
- Hold this position for a short period of time (e.g., 5-15 seconds or more) using an isometric hold approach or raise up for 2 seconds then lower for 2 seconds to complete one repetition
- Maintain neutral head and neck alignment with your body at all times

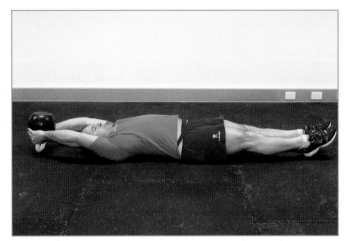
Start

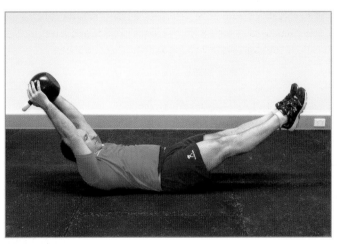
Mid-point

Note: To avoid any arching of the lower back whilst developing core-strength, start with one leg bent and raise the upper body and single leg up and hold. Vary which leg is raised in each set before progressing onto double leg raise a shown.

68. Fitness Ball Crunch Series: Levels 1–3

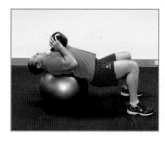
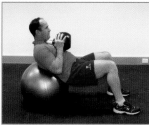

Level 1: Start & Raised

Level 2: Start & Raised

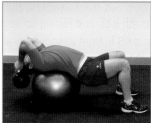
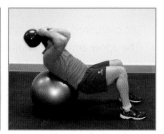

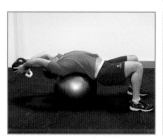
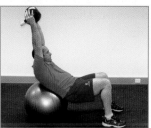

Level 3: Start & Raised

Description

- Lie on your back on a fitness ball with your knees bent and feet resting on the ground, shoulder-width apart with the following arm positions:
  - Level 1 (easy – short lever): Arms across chest, holding a single KB
  - Level 2 (moderate – mid-lever): Arms bent, a single KB resting on its head
  - Level 3 (hard – long lever): Arms extended overhead holding a single KB around its belly
- Apply the 3Bs Principle™
- While breathing out, contract the abdominal muscles and slowly contract and curl the stomach muscles up, bringing the sternum toward the pelvis
- Breathe in and lower
- Maintain the head in its neutral position throughout the exercise to avoid neck tension
- Aim to curl and raise up for 2 seconds and lower for 2 seconds to complete one repetition

69. Collins-Lateral KB Fly™

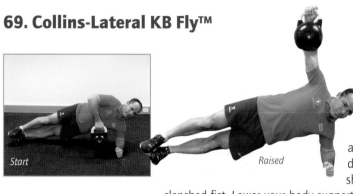

Start   *Raised*

Description
• Lie on your side with your upper body supported by an elbow (90 degrees, directly below the shoulder), forearm and clenched fist. Lower your body supported by your feet, which are positioned together along with legs, and resting on edge of your shoe

• The upper arm is bent holding a KB in front of your body across the chest area and close to a supporting hand on the ground

• Lift the pelvis off the ground, eliminating the side bending by rising onto the edge of your shoes, forming a straight line from the feet to head

• Apply the 3Bs Principle™

• Maintaining a deep breathing pattern, raise the upper arm in a semi-circular motion until vertical then lower to complete one repetition

• Repeat drill on the opposite side

Variation
• Raise your upper leg to increase the challenge while lowering and raising your arm

70. Fitness Ball Oblique Twist

Start

Description
• Lie on a fitness ball at shoulder height with your hips raised and body parallel to the ground. Your feet are shoulder-width apart, arms are extended above the chest, gripping the outer handles of KBs in both hands

• Apply the 3Bs Principle™

• Keep the arms in line with the upper body and slowly twist the arms and shoulders across to the left side. At the same time, bend at the knees and rotating the hips and torso with your left shoulder rising onto the ball. Arms are parallel to the ground

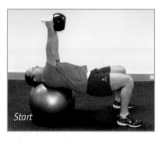

Mid-point

• Keeping the arms extended, rotate a KB across the body to the right side, up onto the right shoulder with your arms once again parallel to the ground

• Move your head in time with your body and in line with the shoulder in neutral position. Twist slowly under tension for 3 seconds on each side

71. KB Isometric Twist

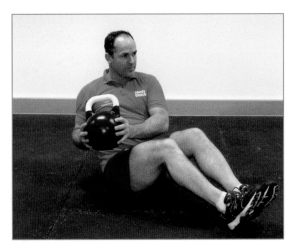

Start

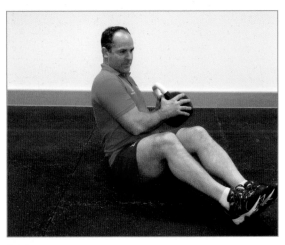

Rotate

Description

- Sit on the ground with your body at approximately a 45-degree angle with your legs extended and slightly bent. Arms are extended forward holding the belly of a single KB in both hands
- Apply the 3Bs Principle™
- Maintaining a constant breathing pattern, with the abdominals braced and shoulders square move the KB from side to side (just outside the line of knee) using only the arms, in a controlled manner for a set amount of time or repetitions
- This movement primarily uses the arms and limits any body rotation or lower back twisting to avoid overuse or stress

Variations

- Raise both feet off the ground and hold your abdominals tight
- Advanced: Grip the handle with both hands and keeping your wrists straight, twist the KB across your body avoiding any lower back stress

72. KB Overhead Walk

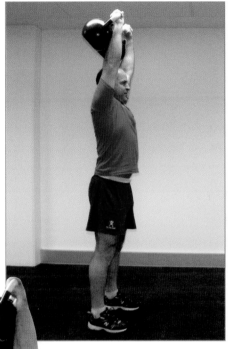

Start

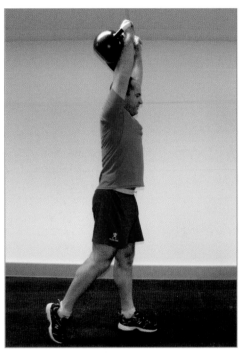

First step

The abdominopelvic cavity also plays an important role in bracing and holding good posture in various physical activities by helping stabilize the spine. The KB Overhead Walk is a postural development drill for strengthening the abdominal region through the application of the 3Bs Principle™.

- Start with both your arms extended overhead, gripping KBs in both hands
- Apply the 3Bs Principle™
- Walk forward over a set distance while ensuring good posture and arm position over your head. Focus on core positioning at all times

Note: This exercise is focused on the abdominal brace. Having the KBs held overhead and walking challenges the abdominal brace. If the bracing is lost, the exercise needs to be stopped

Continue walking forward

CHAPTER 4
Stage 2: Swing Pattern

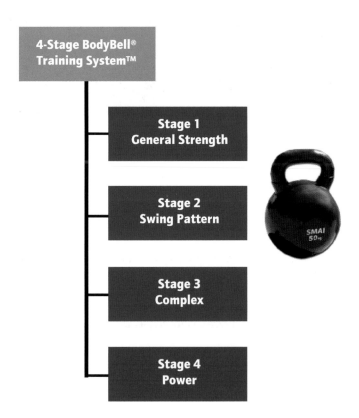

**4-Stage BodyBell®
Training System™**

**Stage 1
General Strength**

**Stage 2
Swing Pattern**

**Stage 3
Complex**

**Stage 4
Power**

SMAI
50kg

73. Double Arm Front Swing

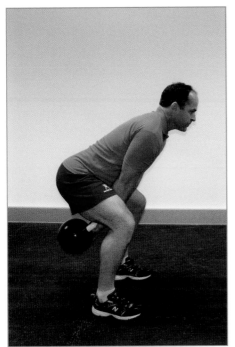

Start

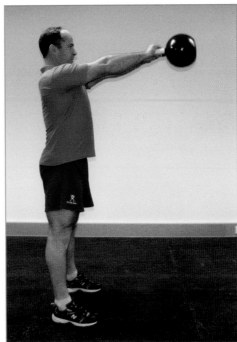

Mid-point

Description
- Stand with your feet wider than shoulder-width, legs bent in squat position, back flat, head forward and arms extended down, gripping a KB with both hands (knuckles forward)
- Apply the 3Bs Principle™
- Simultaneously rise from the squat position while swinging your arms forward. It may take you 2-3 swings to reach the required swing height. (For swing arc ranges, refer to Swing Arm Arc Range in Chapter 2)
- At the top of the arm movement, tighten your abdominal muscles and glutes before lowering back down to squat position. Maintain good muscle control and sequencing at all times

74. Single Arm Front Swing

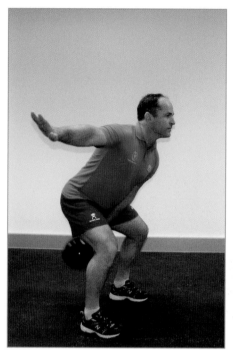

Start

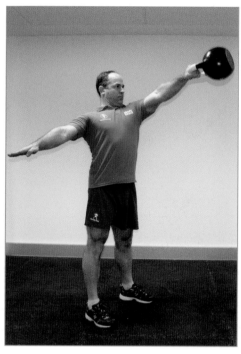

Mid-point

Description

- Stand with your feet wider than shoulder-width, legs bent in squat position, back flat, head forward and arms extended down, gripping a KB with both hands (knuckles forward)
- Apply the 3Bs Principle™
- Simultaneously rise from the squat position while swinging your arms forward. It may take you 2-3 swings to reach the required swing height. (For swing arc ranges, refer to Swing Arm Arc Range in Chapter 2)
- At the top of the arm movement with hip extended, tighten your abdominal muscles and glutes before lowering back down to the squat position. Maintain good muscle control and sequencing at all times
- Repeat with opposite arm

75. Front Swing Switch Overs

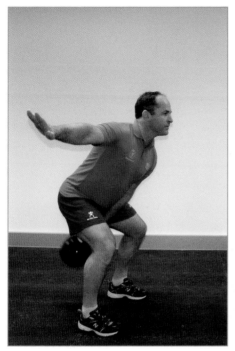

1. Start

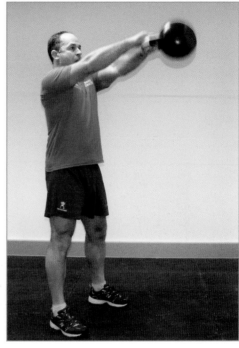

2. Switch

Description
- Stand with your feet wider than shoulder-width, legs bent in squat position, back flat, head forward and arms extended down, gripping a KB with both hands (knuckles forward)
- Apply the 3Bs Principle™
- Simultaneously rise up from the squat position while swinging your arm forward
- At the top of the arm movement, swap hands as you tighten your abdominal muscles and glutes before lowering back down to the squat position. Maintain good muscle control and sequencing at all times
- Repeat the pattern

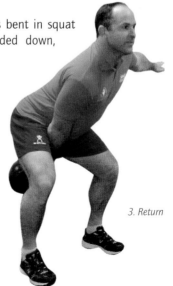

3. Return

76. Double KB Front Swing

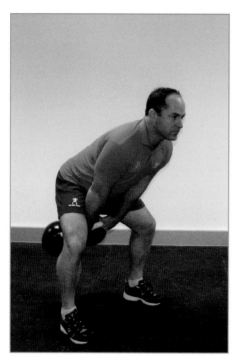

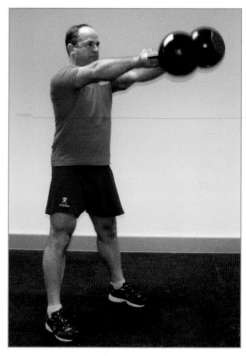

Start

Mid-point

Description
- Stand with your feet wider than shoulder-width, legs bent in squat position, back flat, head forward and arms extended down, gripping two KBs, one in each hand (knuckles forward)
- Apply the 3Bs Principle™
- Simultaneously rise up from the squat position while swinging both arms forward. It may take you 2-3 swings to reach the required swing height
- At the top of the arm movement with hip extended, tighten your abdominal muscles and glutes before lowering back down to squat position. Maintain good muscle control and sequencing at all times
- Repeat the pattern

77. Figure 8s

Description

- Start in a semi-squat position with your feet wider than shoulder-width and arm extended down, holding a KB in front of your body
- Apply the 3Bs Principle™
- Draw the KB across and under the opposite leg. Then swap hands and rotate it around your leg and back across and under the opposite leg to form a figure 8
- Repeat the drill in the opposite direction

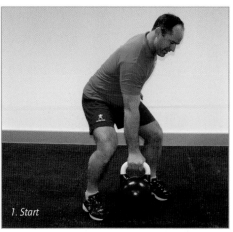

1. Start

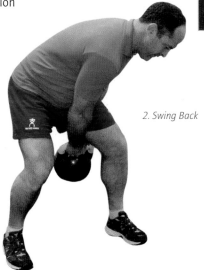

2. Swing Back

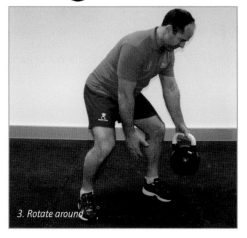

3. Rotate around

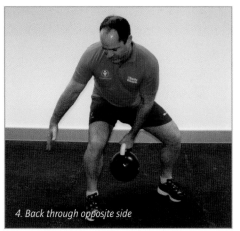

4. Back through opposite side

78. KB Rotations

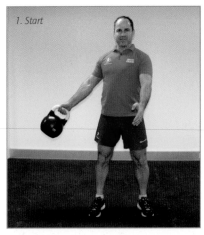

1. Start

Description

- Stand tall with your arm gripping a KB out to the side of your body
- Apply the 3Bs Principle™
- Pull the KB across the body toward your opposite hand
- Catch with your opposite hand and continue to rotate it behind your body
- Take your free behind your body, release the KB and catch
- Continue rotating the KB around your body
- Repeat the drill in the opposite direction

2. Swing across body

4. Back around to front

3. Around back

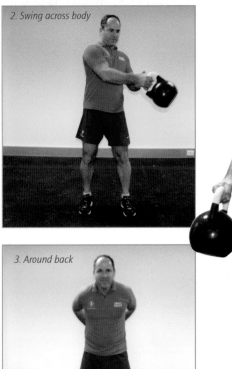

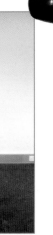

79. KB Side Swing

1. Start wide

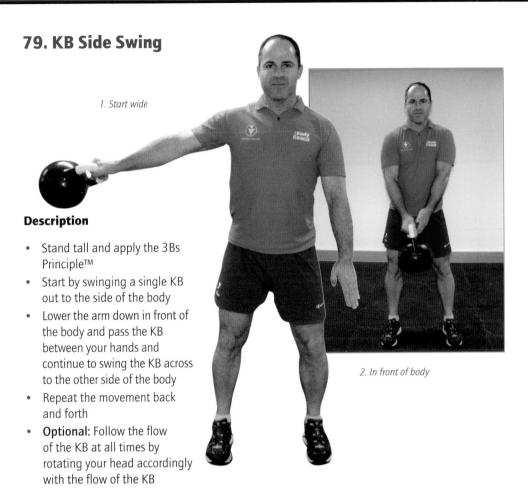

2. In front of body

Description

- Stand tall and apply the 3Bs Principle™
- Start by swinging a single KB out to the side of the body
- Lower the arm down in front of the body and pass the KB between your hands and continue to swing the KB across to the other side of the body
- Repeat the movement back and forth
- **Optional:** Follow the flow of the KB at all times by rotating your head accordingly with the flow of the KB

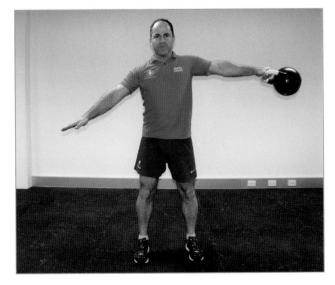

3. Across to opposite side

80. KB Side Swing

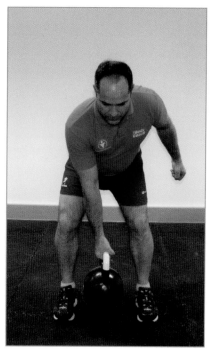

Start

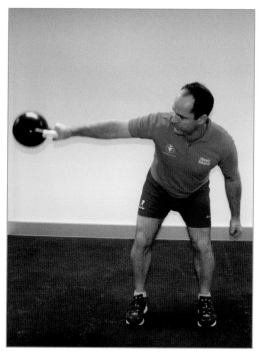

Mid-point

Description
- Stand in a semi-squat position with the torso in front of the knee line and an arm extended down, gripping a KB in front of the body. The opposite arm is by your side
- Apply the 3Bs Principle™
- Swing the arm out to the side and back in a controlled motion, keeping the wrist straight at all times
- Repeat with the opposite arm
- **Optional:** Follow the flow of the KB at all times by rotating your head accordingly with the flow of the KB

CHAPTER 5
Stage 3: Complex KB Exercises

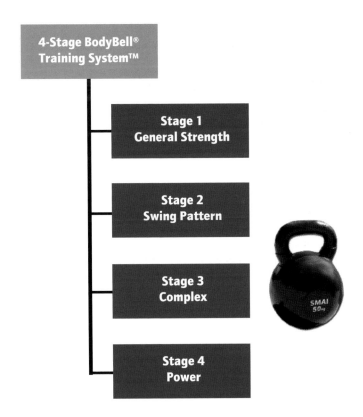

4-Stage BodyBell®
Training System™

Stage 1
General Strength

Stage 2
Swing Pattern

Stage 3
Complex

Stage 4
Power

81. Basic Bent Press

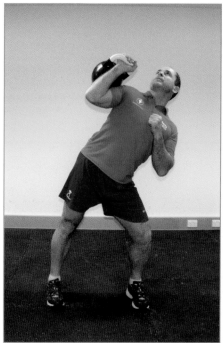

Start

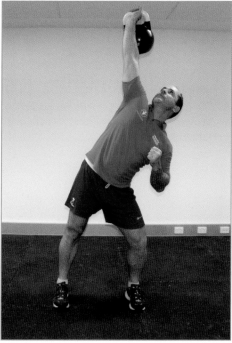

Mid-point

Description:
- Start by holding a single KB in the rack position with your feet shoulder-width apart
- Step forward with the opposite leg of the lifting arm and slightly turn the foot on the lifting side
- Push the hip on the lifting side out, locking the leg out while the opposite leg is slightly bent and the foot is pointing straight forward
- Depending on your flexibility:
  - Position your forearm vertically and to the side of your ribcage, turning the opposite shoulder away in order to do this
  - From rack position, hold the KB in a balanced position above the shoulder (as shown)
- Raise and lower your arm from this position
- Repat on the opposite side

82. Side Press

Description:

- Start by holding a single KB in the rack position with your feet shoulder-width apart
- Step forward with the opposite leg as the lifting arm and slightly turn the foot on the lifting side
- Push the hip on the lifting side out, locking the leg out while the opposite leg is slightly bent and the foot is pointing straight forward
- Depending on your flexibility:
  - Position your forearm vertically and to the side of your ribcage, turning the opposite shoulder away in order to do this
  - From rack position, hold the KB in a balanced position above the shoulder (as shown)
- Slowly lean forward and lower your body away from the KB, keeping your eyes on the KB throughout the whole movement
- As you lean, simultaneously raise the arm in a natural, balanced movement while lowering the opposite arm toward the ground, forming one line from the ground up to the KB before moving your body back up and the KB to rack position
- Repeat on the opposite side

Advanced athlete's progression:

Once your arm is straight, bend both legs (keeping your eyes on the KB) and lower down into an overhead squat position. Rise up, pressing your weight through your heels, keeping the arm locked out. Upon standing, lower the KB back into the rack position.

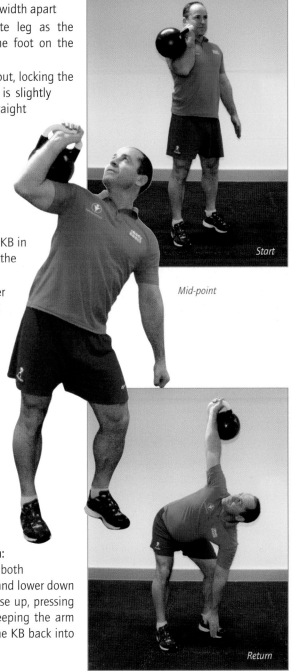

Start

Mid-point

Return

83. Basic Windmill

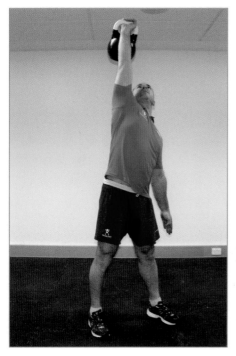
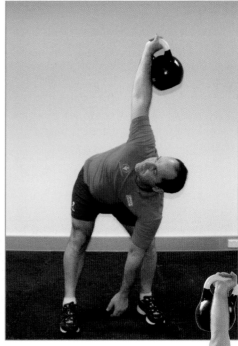

Start

2. Lowered

Description
- Clean and press the KB to an overhead position while standing tall with your feet turned out at a slight angle. Your eyes should be focused on the KB overhead
- Slowly bend at the hips, keeping most of your weight on the heel of the foot of the raised arm, and continue to move your hip backwards and to the side with the KB remaining vertical
- Lower your upper body toward the ground until reaching your range of motion (without stress or pain), then drive through your hips and stand back up squeezing your glutes
- Repeat with the opposite arm

Caution: This exercise is for advanced athletes only as it requires great control and flexibility with stability. Do not attempt this exercise if you have suffered any previous lower back stress, tension or injury. Always perform exercises under the guidance of a strength and conditioning coach.

Variation
- Hold two KBs to perform the Double Windmill

Raised

84. Single Arm High Pull

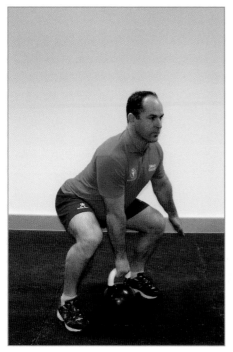

Start

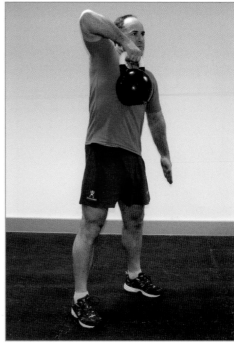

Mid-point

Description
- Start in a squat position with your feet wider than shoulder-width, one arm extended down, gripping a KB that is resting on the ground (knuckles forward). The other arm is out by your side
- Apply the 3Bs Principle™
- Simultaneously power up off ground through the legs, rising up onto your toes, while raising your elbow up high with the KB before lowering it in a controlled motion
- Repeat the drill using the opposite arm

Variation
- Swing High Pull – with arc (KB is swinging up in front)

85. Single Arm Squat Press

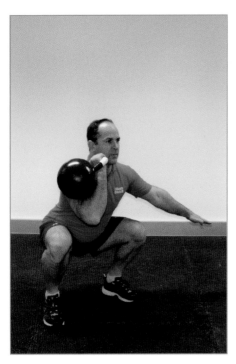

Lowered

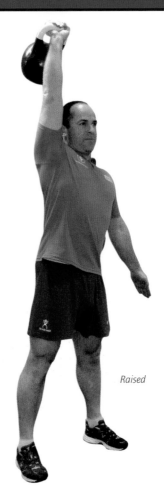

Raised

Description
- Stand with your feet shoulder-width apart, one arm gripping a KB in the rack position, and the other arm extended out to your side
- Apply the 3Bs Principle™
- Breathe in as you squat down until your thighs are parallel to the ground. Bend at the hips, knees and ankles while keeping the KB in rack position
- Breathe out as you reverse the movement and rise up while extending the arm up overhead with the KB
- Breathe in again as you lower back down to squat position, bringing the KB back to the rack position before repeating the movement for your desired number of repetitions
- Repeat the drill with the KB in the opposite hand

86. Push Press – Single KB

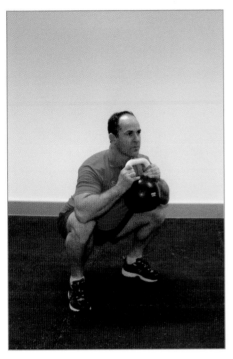

Start

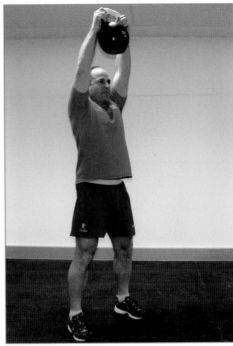

Mid-point

Description
- Stand tall with your feet shoulder-width apart and your arms bent in front of your body, with both hands holding a KB at chest height
- Apply the 3Bs Principle™
- Breathe in as you simultaneously squat down until the thighs parallel to the ground. Bend at the hips, knees and ankles while keeping the KB against your chest
- Breathe out as you rise while extending the arms up overhead with the KB
- Breathe in again as you lower back down to squat position, bringing the KB back to starting position against your chest before repeating the movement for your desired number of repetitions

Variation
- Hand hold position on the KB – handle, bell itself or similar apparatus

87. Push Press – Double KB

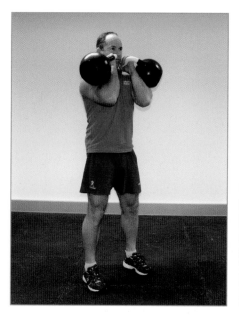

Start

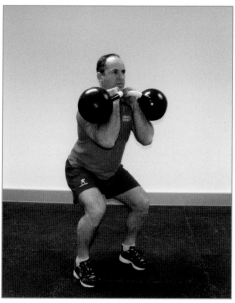

Dip

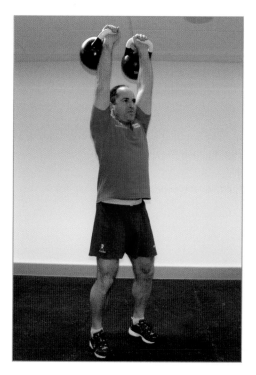

Raised

Description

- Stand tall with your feet shoulder-width apart and your arms bent with KBs held in rack position
- Apply the 3Bs Principle™
- Breathe in as you bend at the hips, knees and ankles while keeping the KBs in rack position before breathing out and simultaneously straightening the legs and extending both arms up and overhead
- Breathe in again as you lower the KBs back into rack position to complete one repetition

88. Get-ups

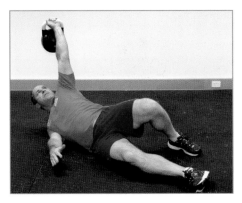

1. Lie

2. Roll

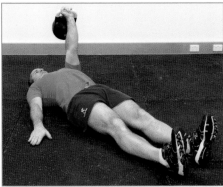

3. Kneel

Description

- Lie on your back with your legs straight and left arm extended vertically holding a KB, palm up
- Apply the 3Bs Principle™
- Keeping the KB arm locked out at all times, roll across onto your right arm triceps and up onto your hand and right thigh
- Keep your eyes on the KB as you continue to push up on the right hand and knee, ensuring the KB remains vertical
- Continue this movement pattern by rising on your knees and up onto both feet with the KB raised vertically overhead
- Take a moment to reset your body position before reversing the movement back to the ground, maintaining full body control while watching the KB and keeping your arms locked out at all times
- Repeat the exercise holding the KB in the opposite hand

4. Stand

89. Hammer Curl to Shoulder Press

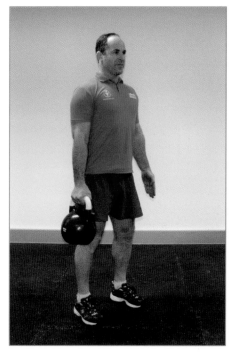

1. Start

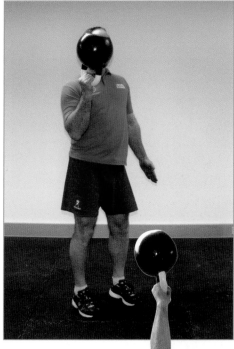

2. Curl

Description

- Stand with your feet shoulder-width apart, one arm extended down by your side, gripping a KB (knuckles out). The other arm is extended out by your side
- Apply the 3Bs Principle™
- Keeping your wrist straight, bend your elbow and curl the KB up to your shoulder with your upper arm held close to your body
- Upon reaching shoulder height, continue the movement by pressing the KB up overhead
- Hold briefly, ensuring a good grip and wrist control before reversing the motion in downward to the starting position to complete one repetition
- Ensure your wrist and forearm remain straight at all times
- Repeat the drill with the opposite arm

3. Press

90. Push up

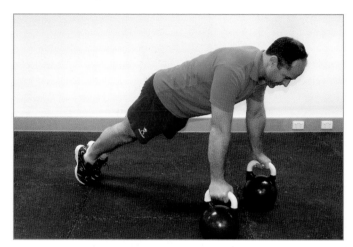

Start

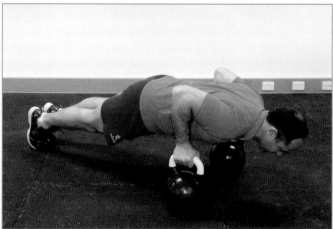

Mid-point

Description

- Position 2 KBs on the ground approximately shoulder-width apart with the handles parallel
- Lower your body into a front support (push-up) position resting on your toes with your feet close together and hands gripping KBs. The arms should be straight and aligned directly over your shoulders
- Apply the 3Bs Principle™
- Breathe in as you lower your chest toward your hands by bending your elbows to an approximate 90-degree angle. Keep your upper arms close to the body and wrists straight
- Breathe out as you rise back up, straightening your arms to complete one repetition

91. Push up to Row

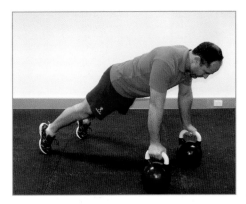

1. Start

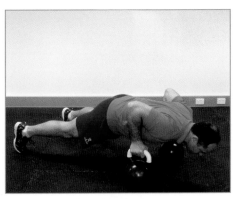

2. Lowe

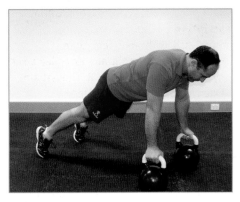

3. Rise

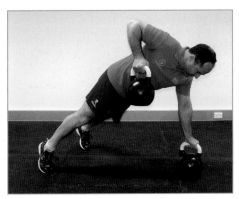

4. Row

Description
- Position 2 KBs on the ground approximately shoulder-width apart with the handles parallel
- Lower your body into a front support (push-up) position resting on your toes with your feet close together and hands gripping KBs. The arms should be straight and aligned directly over your shoulders
- Apply the 3Bs Principle™
- Breathe in as you lower your chest toward your hands by bending your elbows to an approximate 90-degree angle. Keep your upper arms close to the body and wrists straight
- Breathe out as you rise back up, straightening your arms while simultaneously performing a one-armed row, then lower the KB back to the starting position to complete one repetition.
- Repeat the movement, performing the row with the opposite arm

92. Stationary Lunge Cross-overs

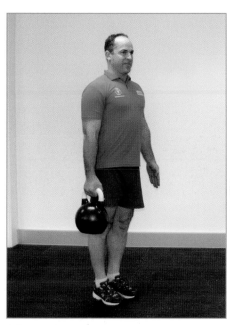

2. Mid-point

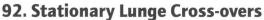

1. Start

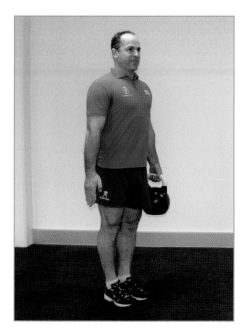

3. Return

Description

- Stand tall with your feet close together and the right arm extended down by your side, gripping a KB. The left arm is extended out to side for balance
- Apply the 3Bs Principle™
- Breathe in as you lunge forward with the left leg until the front thigh is parallel to the ground (knee over the toes) and the rear knee is close to the ground. At the same time, pass the KB under your legs and swap hands, while ensuring the torso remains as upright as possible
- Breathe out as you push back up off the front leg to the upright starting position to complete one repetition with the KB now held in the opposite hand
- Repeat the drill by lunging forward with the opposite leg

Variations

- Stationary Lunge Crossover
- Continuous crossovers – lunge forward in a continuous walking motion

93. Lunge Press – Single KB

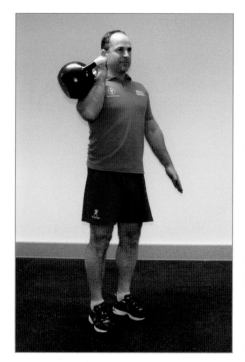

Start

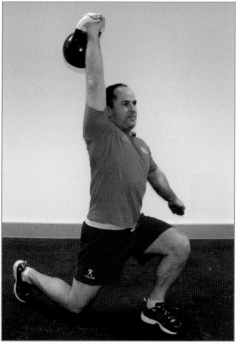

Mid-point

Description
- Stand tall with your feet close together, your right hand holding a KB in rack position and your left arm extended out to the side
- Apply the 3Bs Principle™
- Lunge forward with your left leg, lowering your rear knee toward the ground while pushing the right arm with the KB overhead
- Push back off your leading leg to an upright starting position while returning the KB to rack position
- Repeat the drill on the opposite side

Variation
- Start in a stationary lunge position and, as you lower your knee, raise your arm

94. Lunge Press – Double KB

Description
- Stand tall with your feet together and KBs resting in front of your body at shoulder height.
- Apply the 3Bs Principle™
- While breathing in, simultaneously raise your arms up overhead while stepping forward with one leg into a lunge position. The front thigh is parallel to the ground and the knee is over your toes
- Breathe out as you rise back up to starting position and return your arms to rest the KBs at shoulder height to complete one repetition
- Repeat the drill with the opposite leg lunging forward

Variations
- Both hands above your head at all times
- Constant forward walking lunge movement
- Lunging forward, diagonally, laterally and backwards
- Lunging with your lateral arm raised from the side of the body and other multiple arm movement positions for a challenge

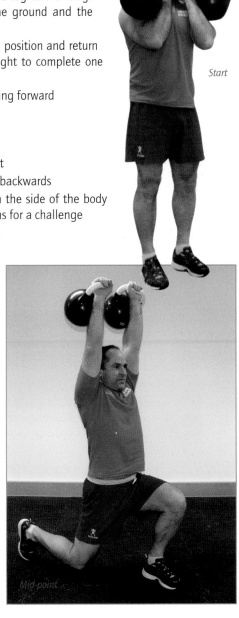

Start

Mid-point

This exercise aims to strengthen the glutes, hamstrings, legs and shoulders with a focus on core control

Note: See Stationary Lunge Starting Position (page 75) for alternate lunge arm configurations, which provide additional challenge opportunities. Use these as the end position with the rear knee lowered when lunging forward from a standing position with your feet starting side by side.

95. Lunge Rotation

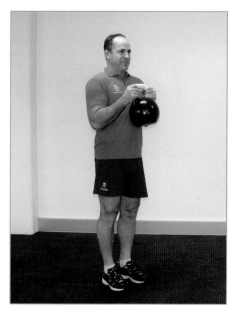
1. Start

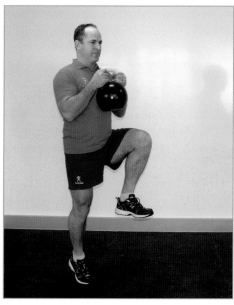
2. Raise Knee

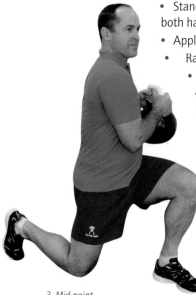
3. Mid-point

Description
- Stand tall with feet together, gripping the outside of a KB handle in both hands against your stomach
- Apply the 3Bs Principle™
- Raise your knee and lunge forward with your left leg
  - Land in a controlled motion, keeping your torso upright
  - Rotate the KB across your body to the left side and back before pushing off your front leg back up to starting position
  - Repeat the drill on your right leg, keeping the KB close to the body at all times when rotating
    - his exercise aims to strengthen the glutes, hamstrings, legs and abdominals with a focus on good core control

Variation
- This exercise can also be performed in a forward motion, continually lunging forward for 10 steps or more while rotating the KB across the body.

96. Squat to Lunge

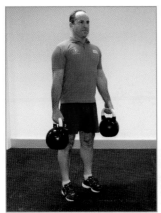
1. Start

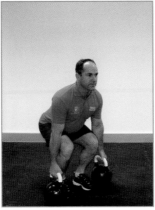
2. Squat

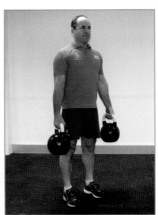
3. Rise

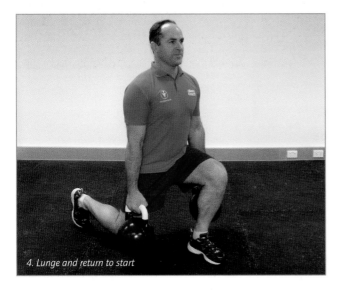
4. Lunge and return to start

Description
- Stand tall with your feet hip-width apart, gripping KBs at arm's length by your sides, knuckles facing out
- Apply the 3Bs Principle™
- Breathe in as you squat down until your thighs are parallel by pushing back through the hips, knees and ankles
- Breathe out as you rise up to starting position
- Breathe in again as you lunge forward with your left leg, bending the front knee until the thigh is parallel to the ground with your knees aligned over your toes and the rear knee lowered toward the ground. Your arms remain by your sides
- Breathe out as you push back up off the left leg and return the body back up to the upright starting position to complete one repetition
- Repeat the squat and forward lunge with the right leg

Variation
- Hands can be held in the rack position throughout. In addition, if in the rack position, press both hands overhead when lunging forward.

97. Triceps Press to Chest Fly

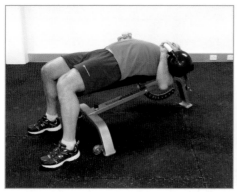

1. Start

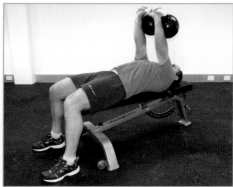

2. Press

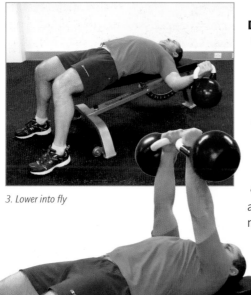

3. Lower into fly

4. Chest Fly

Description

- Lie on your back on a flat weight bench with your knees bent and your feet on the ground shoulder-width apart. Your arms are bent with KBs held close to the body at chest height
- Apply the 3Bs Principle™
  - Breathe out as you press both arms directly up to full extension and close together, keeping your wrists straight
  - From the top, breathe in as you lower your arms out wide to the sides in a semi-circular motion while your rotating hands and maintaining a slight bend in the arms as you lower them down to chest height
  - Breathe out again as you raise your arms back up again in a semi-circular motion, keeping your arms slightly bent at all times until the KBs come together overhead
  - Rotate your hands as you lower back down to the original start position to complete one repetition

Variation

- This exercise targets the chest and triceps muscles and can also be performed on a fitness ball with the assistance of a qualified strength and conditioning coach.

98. Single Arm Fitness Ball Chest Press

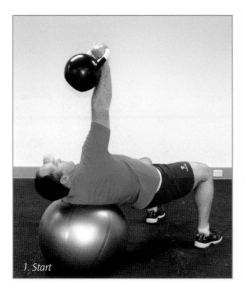

1. Start

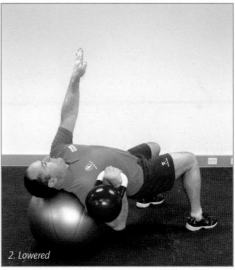

2. Lowered

Description

- Lie on your back with your shoulders on a fitness ball. Your feet should be resting shoulder-width apart on the ground for support. One arm should be extended vertically, holding a KB, palms up, and shoulder raised with a KB over your eye-line while the other arm should be extended out to the side for balance

- Apply the 3Bs Principle™

- Breathe in as you lower the KB while simultaneously rolling your shoulders across the fitness ball, bending the elbow until the KB is level with your chest. Be sure your core is held strong and to extend your free arm overhead for balance

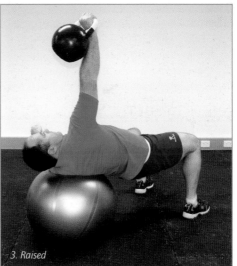

3. Raised

- Breathe out as you press the KB back up overhead, rolling your shoulders slightly across the ball. Raise your shoulders while returning the unweighted arm back by your side at shoulder level to complete one repetition

- Complete the set and repeat with the opposite arm

Variation

- Alternate Arm KB Chest Press

99. Alternate Arm Chest Press

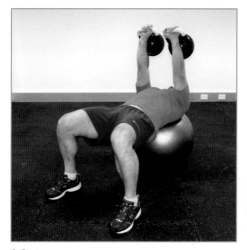
1. Start

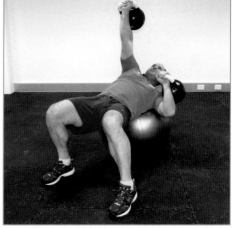
2. Right Arm Press

Description
- Lie on your back and shoulders on a fitness ball with feet resting on ground shoulder-width apart for support and both arms extended directly overhead above your chest, gripping KBs
- Apply the 3Bs Principle™
- Simultaneously rotate your shoulder across the fitness ball as you lower one arm down toward your chest, allowing your waist to rotate to allow for an effective movement
- With one KB lowered, simultaneously raise this arm back up overhead while lowering the other for an alternate chest press

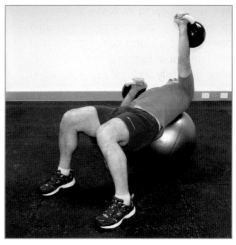
3. Left Raise Press

Variation
- This exercise targets the chest, triceps and core control and can also be performed with one arm lowering and rising back up before lowering the other.

CHAPTER 6
Stage 4: Power Development

Exercise Progression and Technique

Stage 3 Power training provides a series of Olympic lifting-based exercise drills using KBs that help establish strength, speed and technique that ultimately lead to developing explosive power and control. In this stage, a rapid development of force contributes to the development of further speed and power while gradually acclimatizing the central nervous system (CNS). As described in the Foundational Strength Training Zones chart, good technique is the first priority, so it is important to use lighter KBs before increasing the weight and developing more explosive movements.

It is much wiser to have an athlete learn the lifting progressions in order to coordinate, master and perform the movement pattern before putting it all together with more advanced Olympic lifts using KBs. This approach helps speed up the learning curve and make certain that the athlete establishes good technique, neuromuscular coordination and power. The progression element is critically important because along the way your body will have improved its core strength, mobility and neuromuscular capacity. You will have also exposed the connective tissues, tendons, ligaments and muscle fibers to various angles and degrees of resistance and speed, all of which help the body become more functional in sport and allow it to cope with a variety of forces and activities, while also reducing one's risk of injury.

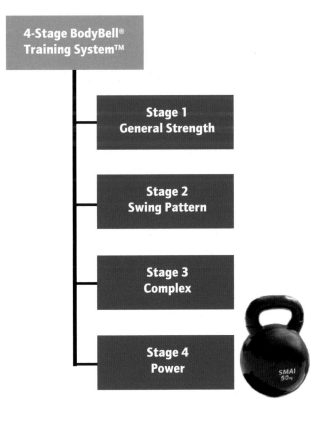

4-Stage BodyBell® Training System™

Stage 1
General Strength

Stage 2
Swing Pattern

Stage 3
Complex

Stage 4
Power

As more complex KB exercises are introduced, you'll feel a greater demand by the Central Nervous System (CNS) in performing each exercise. The strength gains from previous training stages are now being placed through a conversion process where a higher power output is required. The exercises themselves are becoming more complex and sports specific in many ways.

Developing Explosive Power

To perform the lifts encountered in this chapter, you must have successfully progressed through training stages 1 and 2. When learning an Olympic lift using KBs, it is essential that emphasis is placed on learning proper technique first using lighter weights. The goal is to increase power output, which comes from moving a weight quickly. If the weight is too heavy, the KBs will move slowly and the athlete's technique will suffer, potentially causing injury. Over time, as technique and speed improves, gradually the KB weight may be increased, which will contribute to the effective development of speed and power conversion.

As a coach, I understand the importance and benefits of Olympic lifting and the carry-over of better coordination and the development of a higher rate of force to one's sport. Even if that ranges from the traditional power clean to the much more complex snatch, Olympic lifts train the athlete to explode and use the maximum force possible. As a result, quality of movement is favored over quantity with longer rest breaks to ensure the body is fresh when performing lifts.

Power Output Stages

Upon reaching this point in strength training, we see a rapid increase in the power output incurred in each lift. This requires a two-phase approach:

- **Power Phase 1:** Light load (or weight) being lifted at high speed, including medicine balls and Olympic lifts; ensuring mastery of technique; lift speed often used to imitate sport-specific power performed at high velocity, such as the shot put
- **Power Phase 2:** Heavy load being lifted at high speed

Because of the rapid movements and muscle recruitment of these powerful lifts, the nervous system is highly taxed, requiring longer recovery periods of 3-5 minutes between sets. In-between sets, light cardiovascular exercise (i.e., stationary bike) can be performed to assist in feeding oxygen to the working muscles while also assisting later in the cooling down phase followed by stretching to reduce muscle soreness.

Olympic Lifting Stretching Routine

Olympic Lifting requires tremendous strength, mobility and stability of a joint to ensure correct movement technique is maintained at all times. On some occasions, special attention may need to be applied regularly to ensure this mobility is maintained. The following stretches target specific muscular groups utilized in Olympic Lifts. Each stretch is held for up to 15 seconds or more and is repeated on both sides of the body, as required. Meanwhile, for those with excessive range of motion in one joint or a series of joints (commonly referred to as hypermobility) a stability-based approach is required, as opposed to stretching, for better muscle control.

Key Stretches	Description

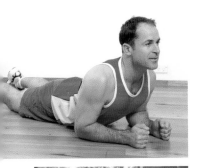

Back extension – elbows
Objective: Stretch lower back muscles, to assist with set-up and first pull phases.

Lie on ground on stomach and forearms and gently raise chest up off ground and hold without stress or pain.

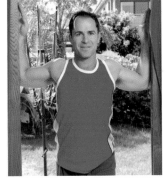

Chest stretch
Objective: Stretch chest muscles and assist in good body alignment, pulling movement and dumbbell position, especially when overhead.

Stand between door frame (or corner of two walls – L-shape) with arms at 90 degrees and gently lean forwards.

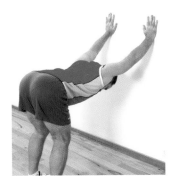

Mid-Back Arch
Objective: Stretch mid and upper back and shoulder region to assist with the dumbbell position, especially when overhead.

Stand opposite to wall and between door frame (or corner of two walls – L-shape). Bend at hips, place hands on wall and gently lean forwards.

Triceps

Objective: Stretch upper back, scapula and triceps important in shoulder and scapula mobility in all upper body and overhead movements.

Bend arms behind head and grip elbow with opposite hand. Gently pull downwards. Repeat with opposite arm.

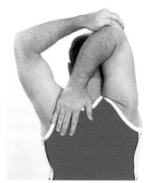

Adductors

Objective: Stretch groin region to assist with rapid leg movement from bent to raised position.

Sit on ground with soles of feet together and place forearms along legs, gripping ankles with hands. Gently push knees down towards grounds by using your arms, before relaxing.

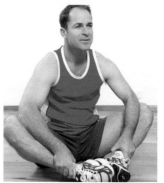

Hamstrings

Objective: Stretch hamstrings muscles involved in squat and lunge movements.

Sit on ground with legs extended and one foot on top of the other. Extend arms behind the body with fingers cupped and pointed. Keeping spine long gently lean forwards for stretch. Repeat with opposite leg.

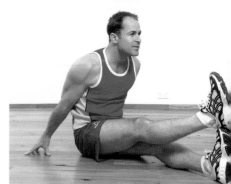

Hip and Thoracic

Objective: Stretch hip and mid back region to ensure pliability of muscle for all movements.

Sit on ground with soles of feet together and place forearms along legs, gripping ankles with hands. Gently push knees down towards grounds by using your arms, before relaxing.

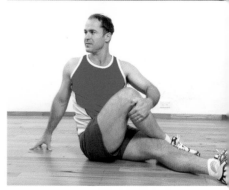

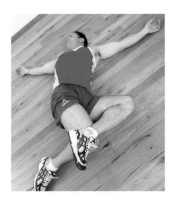

Lumbar rotation
Objective: Stretch hip, lower and mid back regions to ensure pliability of muscle for all movements.

Lie on ground with arms out wide and one leg bent across the other. Lower leg to side and face head across to other side. Repeat opposite direction.

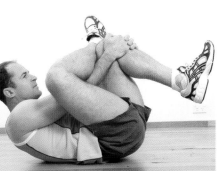

Piriformis
Objective: Stretch deep gluteal muscles involved in all lower body movements.

From the above stretch, lean back onto ground and reach hand of bent leg through hole between legs and the other around outside of leg to both be placed just below knee and pull body close. Repeat opposite leg.

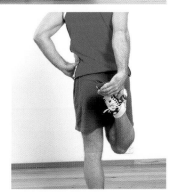

Standing Thigh
Objective: Stretch thigh muscles involved in all squat, lunge and lower body movements.

Standing tall grab foot and bend up behind body and hold. Repeat opposite leg.

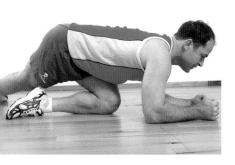

Kneeling sacroiliac joint
Objective: Stretch deep gluteal muscles and sacroiliac joint involved in all lower body movements.

Kneel on ground and lean forwards onto forearms. Cross one leg behind the other keeping the hips square. Repeat opposite leg.

Kneeling hip flexors

Kneeling Side Reach
Objective: Stretch thigh muscles involved in all squat, lunge and lower body movements.

Standing tall, grab foot and bend up behind body and hold. Repeat with opposite leg.

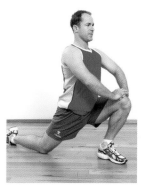
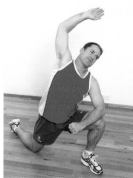

Olympic Lifts

The following exercises are dynamic in nature and require adequate flexibility through the shoulder, back and hip regions to perform correctly. Always practice with light dumbbells first to improve technique and coordination. Apply the 3B's Principle™ - Brace, Breathe and Body Position as part of each Olympic Lift exercise to ensure good quality movement patterns and control at all times. Ensure an appropriate warm-up is undertaken. Always seek professional guidance and one-on-one coaching when undertaking any new exercise.

Note: Due to the forces placed through the feet, ankle and calves in Olympic style lifts, time should also be spent both stretching and strengthening these areas using a stretch and strengthen approach no matter how strong you think your calves are. This includes performing a single calf stretch off the edge of step for 15 seconds followed by 15 single leg calf raises – raising right up onto the ball of the foot and lowering heel down past step. Repeat on both legs.

Jerk

100. One Arm Jerk

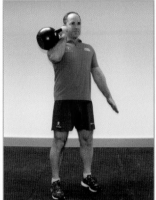
1. Rack

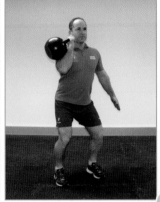
2. Dip

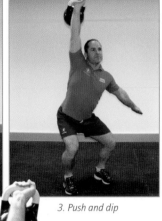
3. Push and dip

Description
- Stand with your feet shoulder-width apart, one hand raised to the side of the body and the other gripping a KB at shoulder height in rack position
- Apply the 3Bs Principle™ -
- Lower into a quarter-squat position before driving back up, raising the arm straight up overhead
- As the arm rises overhead, the legs are dipped again back under the arms to control the KB while standing up straight. Hold the arm extended overhead for 1-3 seconds
- Lower the KB in a controlled motion back into the rack position, absorbing through a slight dip at the knees
- Repeat the drill with the KB in the opposite hand

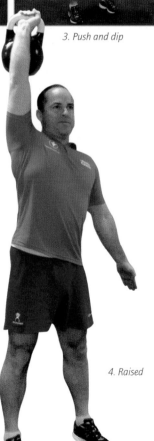
4. Raised

101. One Arm Split Jerk

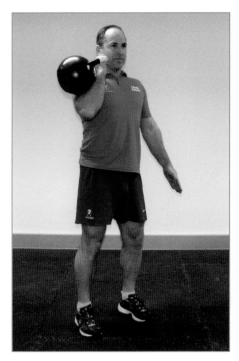
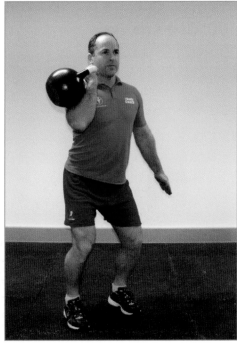

1. Rack   *2. Dip*

Description
- Stand with your feet shoulder-width apart, one hand raised on the side of the body and the other gripping a KB at shoulder height in rack position
- Apply the 3Bs Principle™
- Lower down into a quarter-squat position before driving back up, raising the arm straight up overhead
- As the arm rises overhead, the legs are split (one forward, the other back) into a lunge position under the arm to control the KB
- With the legs split, push off the rear foot forward halfway and bring the front foot back halfway to parallel with the other foot
- Lower the KB in a controlled motion back into the rack position, absorbing the impact with a slight dip at the knees
- Repeat the drill with the KB in the opposite hand

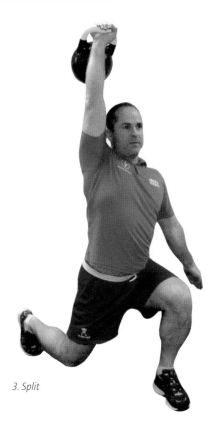

3. Split

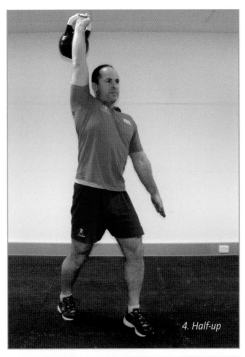

4. Half-up

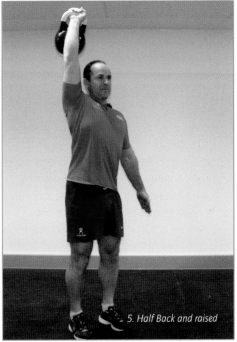

5. Half Back and raised

Note: Some athletes prefer stepping the front foot back first before the rear foot. Do what feels more comfortable to you

102. Double KB Split Jerk

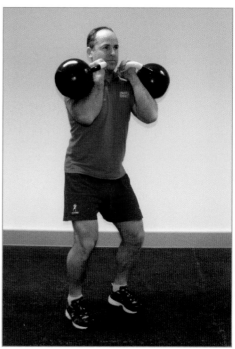

1. Rack

2. Dip

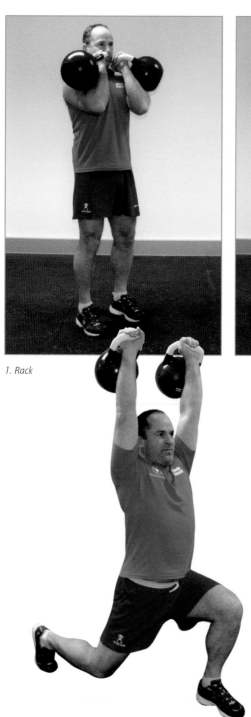

3. Split

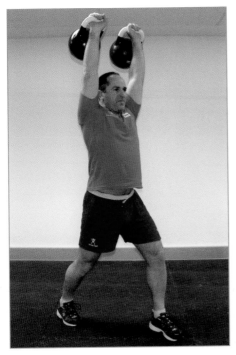

4. Half-up

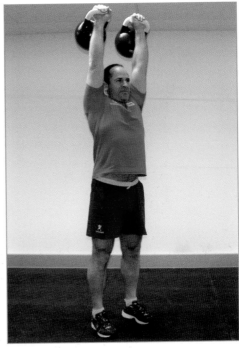

5. Half Back and Raised

Description

- Start with two KBs in the rack position
- Smoothly dip at the hips and knees, keeping the torso straight and vertical before rapidly thrusting up vertically, jumping into a deep split stance. Lock the arms out directly above the head
- Ensure that the KBs travel straight up and that the arm locks out at the top while keeping your torso straight and maintaining good body posture
- Once the KBs are stable above the head and there is good core control, bring the feet back to a parallel stance

Note: A mid-jerk position with less leg bend can also be utilized in the initial strengthening phases

103. Single Arm Push Jerk

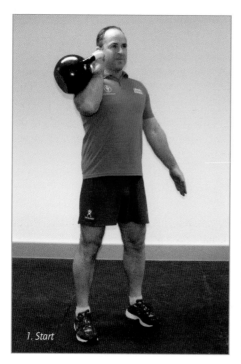
1. Start

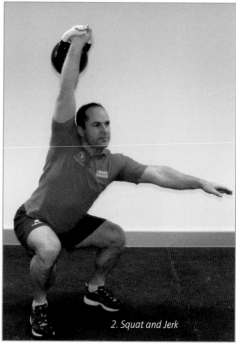
2. Squat and Jerk

Description
- Start with the KB in the rack position and the opposite arm extended by your side
- Allow a brief dip at the hips and knees before rapidly driving your arm overhead to lock out. Lower your body into full squat position, then stand up
- Ensure the arm remains locked directly overhead when lowering and rising the body up to finish

Note: Upon the initial explosive movement, you may jump your feet slightly wider to allow for more effective movement and body control

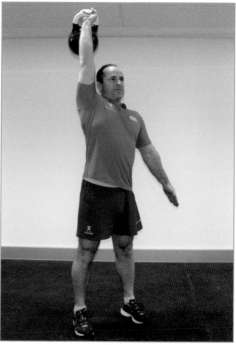
3. Finish

Clean

Hang Position

The hang position is a progressive starting movement for an Olympic-style lift. It is utilized as a progression to movements that may originally start from the ground and in-between drills using a swing motion. This hang movement entails starting in a straight standing position holding a KB or pair of KBs in an extended position in front of the thighs or to the side of the body. This is followed by a dead-lift/squat movement (bending at the hips, knees and ankles) while simultaneously lowering the KB in hand down to:

- slightly above the knee
- slightly below the knee
- toward mid-shin level (just like the start position when using an Olympic bar) followed by the specific pull, clean or snatch motion of an Olympic style lift.

The hang movement illustrated below can be utilized as an added version to many exercises in this section. The KB(s) position itself will vary depending on the specific exercise. Apply accordingly.

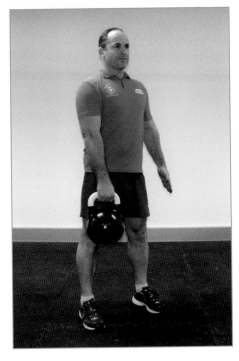

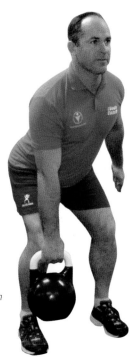

1. Starting Position

2. Hang Position

104. Single Arm Power Clean

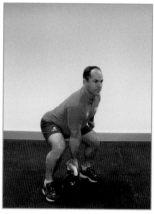
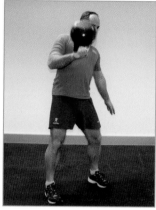
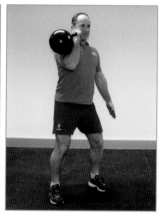

1. Start *2. Pull* *3. Catch in Rack Position*

Description
- Start in a squat position with the KB between your legs and thumb facing backwards
- Drive the body up through extension of the legs, thrusting the hips forward and keeping the KB close to your body
- Maintain the same torso angle during the initial pull phase avoiding the hips rising before or faster than the shoulders
- As the KB reaches near-maximum height, rapidly flex the elbow to bring the body under the KB (elbow tucked into the body and the KB swiveling in hand) into the rack position while absorbing the movement through the legs with a slight dip, then immediately stand up
- Ensure the spine remains neutral and does not round while pulling the KB
- Repeat with the opposite arm

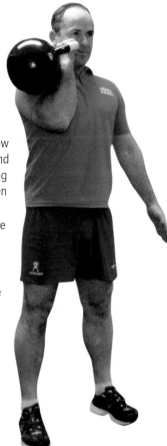

4. Rise

Variations
Hand Grip Start Position
- Thumb sideways, knuckles forward
- Thumb backwards, knuckles inward toward the midline

Start: Ground start; Hang start; Swing start
Rack: Front rack; Side rack
Other: Squat depth; Left and right arm options or both together

105. Cross Body Clean

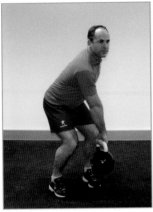
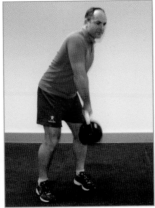
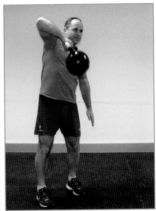

1. Start   *2. Pull*   *3. Catch in Rack Position*

Description
- Start in a semi-squat position with the KB across in front of the opposite knee with thumb facing backwards
- Drive the body up through extension of the legs, thrusting the hips forward. Keep the KB close to your body
- Maintain the same torso angle during the initial pull phase. Be sure the hips don't rise before or faster than the shoulders
- As the KB reaches near maximum height, rapidly flex the elbow to bring the body under the KB (elbow tucked into the body and KB swiveling in hand) into the rack position while absorbing the movement through the legs with a slight dip, then immediately stand up
- Ensure the spine remains neutral and does not round while pulling the KB
- Repeat with the opposite arm

Variations
Hand Grip Start Position
- Thumb sideways, knuckles forward
- Thumb backwards, knuckles inward toward the midline

Start: Ground start; Hang start; Swing start;
Rack: Front rack; Side rack;
Other: Squat depth; Left and right arm options or both together

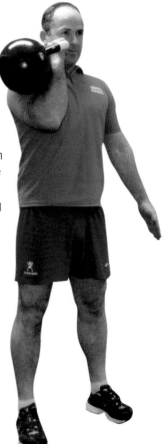

4. Rise

106. Cross Body Snatch

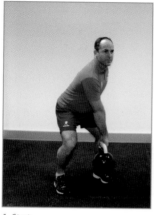
1. Start

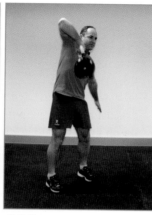
2. Pull

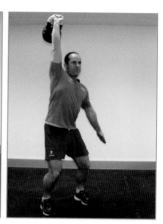
3. Snatch & Catch

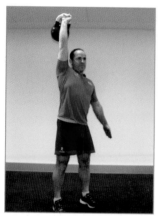
4. Rise

Description

- Start in a semi-squat position with the KB across in front of the opposite knee with the thumb facing backwards
- Drive the body up through extension of the legs, thrusting the hips forward, keeping the KB close to your body
- Maintain the same torso angle during the initial pull phase. Make sure the hips don't rise before or faster than the shoulders.
- As the KB reaches near maximum height, rapidly extend the elbow and hand overhead while bringing the body under the KB. Absorb the movement through the legs with a slight dip, then immediately stand up with the KB extended overhead
- Ensure the spine remains neutral and does not round while pulling the KB
- Repeat with the opposite arm

Variations

Hand Grip Start Position
- Thumb sideways, knuckles forward
- Thumb backwards, knuckles inward toward the midline

Start: Ground start; Hang start; Swing start;
Rack: Front rack; Side rack;
Other: Squat depth; Left and right arm options or both together

107. Single KB Swing Clean

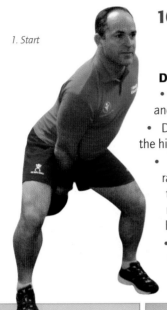

1. Start

Description

- Start in a swing position with the KB between the legs and the opposite arm extended by your side
- Drive the body up through extension of the legs, thrusting the hips forward while swinging the KB up
- As the arm rises up, swivel the KB in your hand and you rapidly flex the elbow to bring the body under the KB (elbow tucked into the body and KB held at shoulder height in a rack position) while absorbing the movement through the legs with a slight dip, then immediately stand up
- Ensure the spine remains neutral and does not round while swinging the KB
- Repeat with the opposite arm

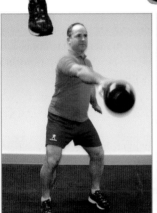
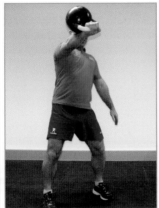
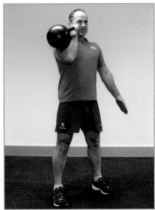

2. Swing   *3. Transition*   *4. Catch and Rack*

Variations

Hand Grip Start Position
- Thumb sideways, knuckles forward
- Thumb backwards, knuckles inward toward the midline

Start: Ground start; Hang start; Swing start;
Rack: Front rack; Side rack;
Other: Squat depth; Left and right arm options or both together

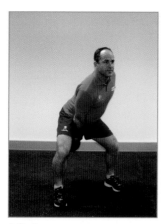

1. Start

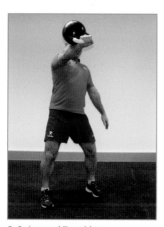

2. Swing and Transition

108. Single KB Swing Squat Clean

Description

- Start in a swing position with the KB between the legs and the opposite arm extended by your side
- Drive the body up through extension of the legs, thrusting the hips forward while swinging the KB up
- As the arm rises up, swivel the KB in your hand and rapidly flex the elbow to bring the body under the KB (elbow tucked into the body and KB held at shoulder height in a rack position) while absorbing the movement through the legs and lowering into a squat position. Then immediately stand up
- Ensure the spine remains neutral and does not round while swinging the KB
- Repeat with the opposite arm

Variations

Hand Grip Start Position
- Thumb sideways, knuckles forward
- Thumb backwards, knuckles inward toward the midline

Start: Ground start; Hang start; Swing start;
Rack: Front rack; Side rack;
Other: Squat depth; Left and right arm options or both together

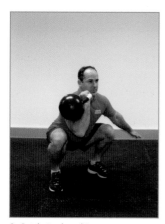

3. Catch, Rack and Squat

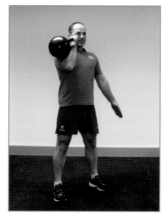

4. Rise

109. Single Arm KB Swing Clean and Jerk

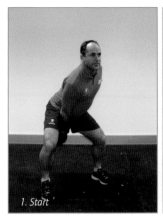

1. Start

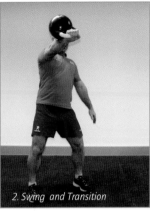

2. Swing and Transition

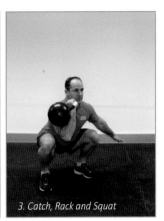

3. Catch, Rack and Squat

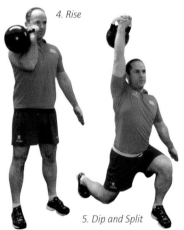

4. Rise

5. Dip and Split

6. Finish

Description

- Start in a swing position with the KB between your legs and the opposite arm extended by your side
- Drive the body up through extension of the legs, thrusting the hips forward while swinging the KB up
- As the arm rises up, swivel the KB in your hand as you rapidly flex the elbow to bring the body under the KB (elbow tucked into the body and KB held at shoulder height in a rack position) while absorbing the movement through the legs and lowering into a squat position. Then immediately stand up
- Ensure the spine remains neutral and does not round while swinging the KB
- Lower down into a quarter-squat position before driving back up, raising the arm straight up overhead
- As the arm rises overhead, the legs are split (one forward, the other back) into a lunge position under the arms to control the KB
- With the legs split, push off the rear foot forward halfway and bring the front foot back halfway to parallel with the feet close together
- Repeat the drill with a KB in the opposite hand

Variation

- Ground start; Hang start; Swing start; Balance arm; Front rack; Side rack; Squat depth; Left and right arm

145

110. Single Arm KB Swing Clean to Press

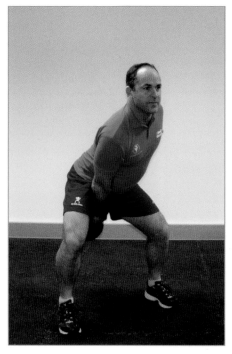

1. Start

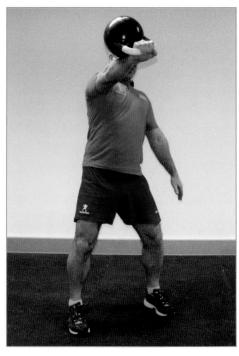

2. Swing and Transition

Description

- Start in a swing position with the KB between your legs and the opposite arm extended by your side
  - Drive the body up through extension of the legs, thrusting the hips forward while swinging the KB up
    - As the arm rises up, swivel the KB in your hand as you rapidly flex the elbow to bring the body under the KB (elbow tucked into the body and KB held at shoulder height in a rack position) while absorbing the movement through the legs and lowering into a squat position. Then immediately stand up
  - Lower down into a quarter-squat position before driving back up, raising the arm straight up overhead
  - As the arm rises overhead, the legs are dipped again back under the arms to control the KB while standing up straight. Hold the arm extended overhead for 1-3 seconds

3. Catch, Rack and Squat

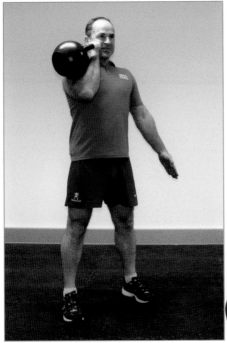

4. Rise

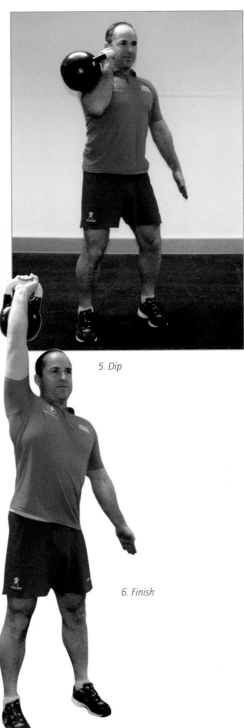

5. Dip

- Lower the KB in a controlled motion back into the rack position, absorbing the movement through a slight dip at the knees
- Repeat the drill with a KB in the opposite hand

Variation
- Ground start; Hang start; Swing start; Balance arm; Front rack; Side rack; Squat depth; Left and right arm

6. Finish

111. Alternating Kettlebell Clean

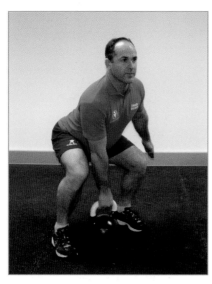

1. Start

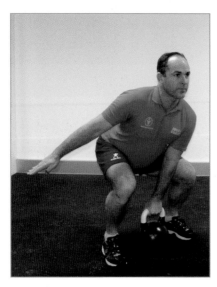

3. Opposite Arm

Description
- Start in a swing position with KB between legs and opposite arm extended by your side
- Drive the body up through extension of the legs, thrusting the hips forward, keeping the KB close to your body
- Maintain the same torso angle during the initial pull phase. Be sure the hips do not rise before or faster than the shoulders
- As the KB reaches near maximum height, rapidly flex the elbow to bring the body under the KB (elbow tucked into the body and KB swiveling in hand) into the rack position while absorbing the movement through the legs with a slight dip, then immediately stand up.
- Lower the KB in a controlled motion back to the ground by bending the knees and repeat the drill with the opposite arm
- Alternate the movement between arms

2. Clean

Variations
Hand Grip Start Position
- Thumb sideways – knuckles forward
- Thumb backwards – knuckles inwards toward midline

Start: Ground start; Hang start; Swing start
Rack: Front rack; Side rack
Other: Squat depth; Left and right arm or both together

112. Double KB Power Clean

Description
- Start in a swing position with KBs between the legs
- Drive the body up through extension of the legs, thrusting the hips forward while swinging the KBs up
- As the arms rise up, swivel the KBs in hand as you rapidly flex the elbows to bring the body under the KBs (elbows tucked into the body and KBs held at shoulder height in a rack position) while absorbing the movement through the legs and lowering into a semi-squat dip position. Then immediately stand up
- Ensure the spine remains neutral and does not round while swinging the KBs

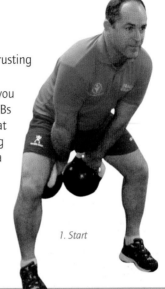

1. Start

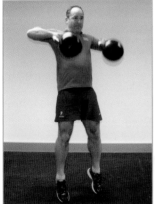

2. Pull

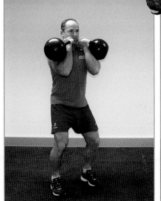

3. Catch

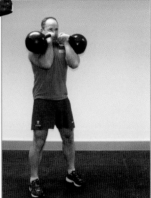

4. Rise

Variations
- Ground start
- Hang start
- Swing start
- Deeper squat catching pattern

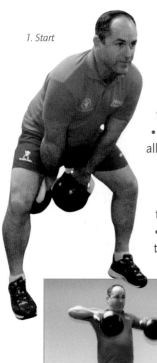

1. Start

113. Double KB Squat Clean

Description

- Start in a semi-squat position with two KBs between your legs
- Drive the body up through extension of the legs, thrusting the hips forward, keeping the KBs close to your body
- Maintain the same torso angle during the initial pull phase. Do not allow the hips to rise before or faster than the shoulders
- As the KB reaches near maximum height, rapidly flex the elbows to bring the body under the KBs (elbows tucked into the body and KBs swiveling in hand) into the rack position while absorbing the movement through the legs with a deep squat. Then immediately stand up
- Ensure the spine remains neutral and does not round while pulling the KBs

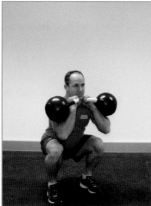
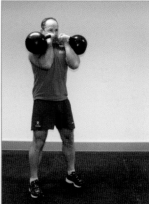

2. Pull   *3. Catch, Rack and Squat*   *4. Rise*

Variations

- Ground start
- Hang start
- Swing start (as shown)

114. Double KB Clean and Jerk

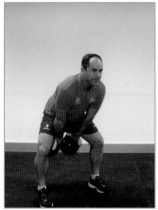

1. Start

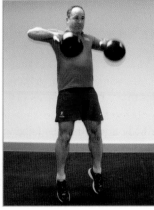

2. Swing and Transition

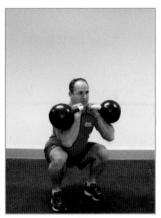

3. Catch, Rack and Squat

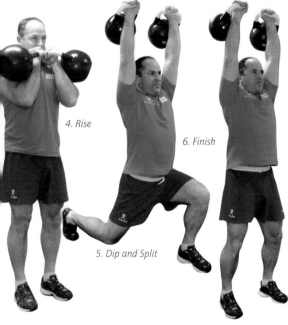

4. Rise

5. Dip and Split

6. Finish

Description

- Start in a semi-squat position with two KBs between your legs
- Drive the body up through extension of the legs, thrusting the hips forward, keeping the KBs close to your body
- Maintain the same torso angle during the initial pull phase. Be sure not to allow the hips to rise before or faster than the shoulders
- As the KB reaches near maximum height, rapidly flex the elbows to bring the body under the KBs (elbows tucked into the body and KBs swiveling in hand) into the rack position while absorbing the movement through the legs with a deep squat. Then immediately stand up
- Ensure the spine remains neutral and does not round while pulling the KBs
- Lower down into a quarter-squat position before driving back up, raising the arms straight up overhead
- As the arm rises overhead, the legs are split (one forward, the other back) into a lunge position under the arms to control the KBs
- With the legs split, push off the rear foot forward halfway and bring the front foot back halfway to parallel with the feet close together

Snatch

115. Single KB Muscle Snatch

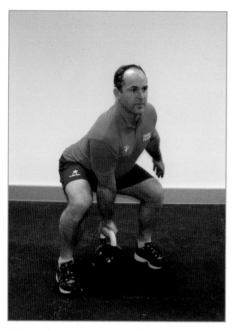

1. Start

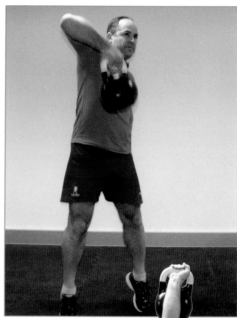

2. Pull

Description
- Start in squat position with one hand gripping the KB between your legs and the other arm extended by your side
- Apply the 3Bs Principle™
- Swing the KB back between the legs, then drive the hips forward allowing the KB to swing out and up
- As the hip drive reaches full extension and the arm is rising, allow the KB to flip around your wrist into an overgrip position resting against your forearm as you punch the arm up, with the KB finishing overhead
- Repeat the drill with the opposite arm

Variations
- Ground start
- Hang start
- Swing start
- Left and right arm
- Double KB versions

3. Catch

116. Single KB Snatch

Description
- Start in squat position with one hand gripping the KB between your legs and the other arm extended by your side
- Apply the 3Bs Principle™
- Swing the KB back between the legs, then drive the hips forward allowing the KB to swing out
  - As the hip drive reaches full extension and the arm is rising, allow the KB to flip around your wrist into an overgrip position resting against your forearm as you punch the arm up, with the KB finishing overhead
    - Stand up with your arm extended holding the KB overhead
    - Repeat the drill with the opposite arm

Variations
- Ground start
- Hang start
- Swing start
- Left and right arm
- Double KB versions

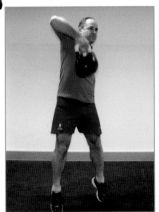

1. Start

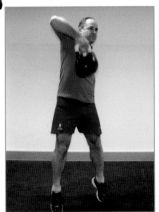

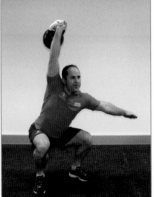

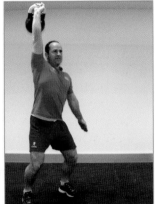

2. Pull   *3. Catch and Squat*   *4. Rise*

117. Double KB Power Snatch

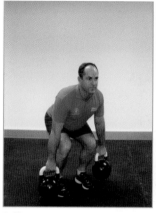
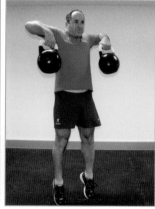
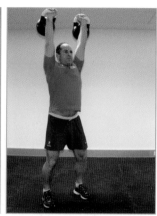

1. Start   2. Pull   3. Catch

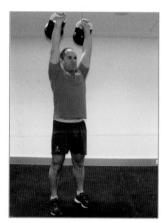

4. Rise

Description
- Start in squat position with KBs positioned at shin height to the side of each leg
- Apply the 3 Bs Principle™
- Drive up through the legs, driving the hips forward and allowing the KBs to swing out and the arms to rise up leading with the elbows
- As the hip drive reaches full extension and the arm is rising, allow the KB to flip around your wrist into an overgrip position resting against your forearm as you punch the arm up, with the KB finishing overhead
- Dip your legs upon catching the KBs on the forearms overhead and before rising

Variations
- Ground start
- Hang start
- Swing start
- Semi-squat with catch (advanced athletes only)

118. Alternating KB Power Snatch

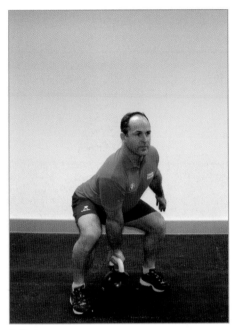

1. Start

2. Catch

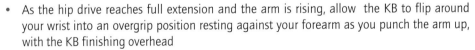

3. Opposite Arm

Description
- Start in squat position with one hand gripping the KB between your legs and the other arm extended by your side
- Apply the 3Bs Principle™
- Drive the body up through extension of the legs, thrusting the hips forward, keeping the KB close to your body
- Maintain the same torso angle during the initial pull phase. Do not allow the hips to rise before or faster than the shoulders
- As the hip drive reaches full extension and the arm is rising, allow the KB to flip around your wrist into an overgrip position resting against your forearm as you punch the arm up, with the KB finishing overhead
- Lower the KB in a controlled motion back to the ground by bending the knees and repeat the drill with the opposite arm
- Alternate the movement between arms

Variations
- Ground start
- Hang start
- Swing start
- Dip and catch

CHAPTER 7
Kettlebell Conditioning Guidelines

Prior to beginning any kettlebell or weight training program, there are a few guidelines you'll need to adhere to:

- Always gain approval to exercise by a medical doctor and physical therapist, especially if you are pregnant or have a previous injury
- See a physical therapist to assess your posture and joint mechanics and to approve appropriate exercises for you
- Have a strength and conditioning coach demonstrate each exercise and correct any faults you may have
- Get to know your muscles in order to understand their function
- It is important during this phase that a proper warm up, cool down and stretching routine is adapted to ensure effective range of motion is maintained and improved
- Stretching is recommended before, during and after exercise, unless a joint or series of joints are hypermobile and require a stability approach. Stretches are short (6 seconds) in nature before and during exercise with a major focus on stretches being held for longer periods (15-30 seconds or more) after training
- If at any time during exercise you feel stress, dizziness, numbness, pain or something similar, stop the exercise and seek appropriate medical advice
- Each exercise should be preceded by a warm-up set using a light resistance band (below 50%) for the specific exercise that follows
- Apply the 3Bs Principle™ with each exercise
- Always maintain good posture and body alignment by focusing on the exercise at hand
- Emphasize quality of movement over quantity
- Maintain deep breathing throughout each exercise. Breathe in on recovery and breathe out when exerting a force, or simply maintain a constant deep breathing pattern at all times
- Never sacrifice your lifting technique for a heavier KB weight
- Rest 60-180 seconds between each set, as required
- Always train under the guidance of a certified strength and conditioning coach, Olympic lifting coach or personal trainer
- Ensure a spotter or trainer is available to help with each exercise as required
- Drink at least two glasses of water during and after your workout
- Give yourself at least 24-72 hours to recover before repeating strength and power training for the same muscle group
- Cool down with light cardiovascular exercise and gentle stretching routine after your workout

Single KB Routine - Sample

Perform appropriate warm-up activities prior to all exercises below

Exercise	Page No.	Reps	Sets	Recovery
1. Sumo Squat				
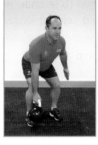 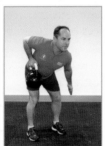	19	10	2-3	60 sec
2. Lineman Row				
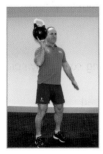 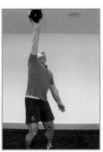	37	12 each arm	2 each arm	60 sec
3. Fingertip Press				
	52	12 each hand	2 each arm	60 sec

Exercise	Page No.	Reps	Sets	Recovery
4. Single leg Deadlift				
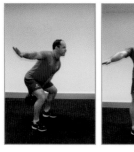 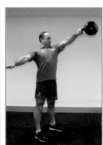	72	10 each leg	2 sets each leg	60 sec
5. Single Arm Front Swing				
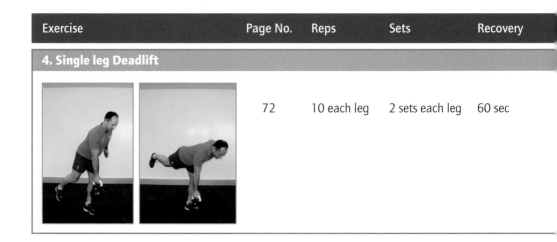	100	10 each arm	2 sets each arm	60 sec
6. KB Sit-Up Rotation				
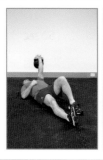 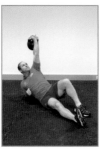	91	10 each arm	2 sets each arm	60 sec

Warm down and stretch upon completion of session

Double KB Routine - Sample

Perform appropriate warm-up activities prior to all exercises below

Exercise	Page No.	Reps	Sets	Recovery
1. Upright Rows – Double KB				
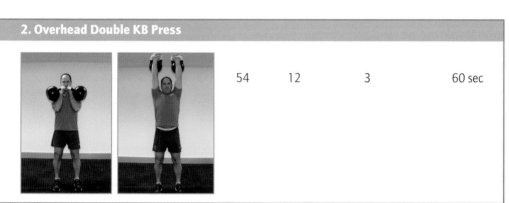	43	12	3	60 sec
2. Overhead Double KB Press				
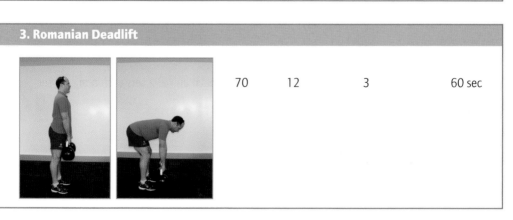	54	12	3	60 sec
3. Romanian Deadlift				
	70	12	3	60 sec

Exercise	Page No.	Reps	Sets	Recovery
4. Alternate Leg Lunge				
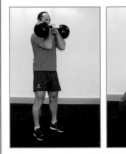	77	12	3	60 sec
5. Front Squat – Double KB Rack Position				
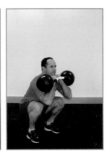	84	12	3	60 sec
6. Double KB Front Swing				
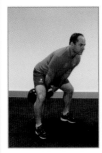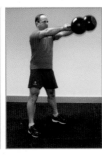	102	12	3	60 sec

Warm down and stretch upon completion of each session

Group Action Drills

Mexican Wave – Extended Arm Space Between Athletes in Large Circle

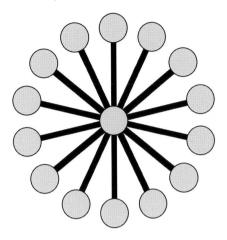

Participants start in a circle, each with plenty of swing space. Using a swing motion, one athlete starts swinging followed shortly after by the person to the right. This progresses in a continuous motion.

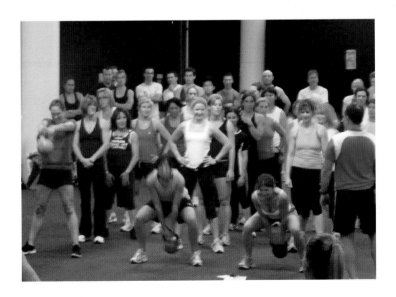

CHAPTER 8
Bonus Section

25 Dynamic Medicine Ball Training Drills

Technology has advanced the production of the old leather medicine ball into a modern air-filled rubber training ball used for dynamic functional movements with a bounce and rebound effect that can be performed against a solid concrete wall, or a tennis, basketball or other ball court and also outdoors on a playing ground for individuals, partners, groups and sport teams.

One of the major benefits of medicine ball training itself is that almost every exercise directly or indirectly conditions the torso (abdominals). A strong torso is essential to every sport, as it provides a stable platform around which the limbs can move effectively, and especially concerning the forces transferred from the legs through to the arms.

There is a vast array of progressive movement patterns and drills in medicine ball training for the mid-section along with the upper and lower extremities used through all planes of movement. Some drills are static and isolated, targeting posture, balance, flexibility, stability and core strength development; while others are more dynamic in nature, involving multiple joints or compound movement patterns via pushing, thrusting and throwing drills for power development, including trapping, catching or further thrusting requirements for eccentric strength development.

Six Developmental Movement Phases

Medicine ball training can be categorized into six important developmental movement phases:

1. General strength exercises involving controlled and mostly isolated exercises on or using a medicine ball, as well as one's own body weight

2. Muscle endurance exercises of medium intensity and higher volume with minimal rest between sets or exercises

3. Concentric-only movements, such as a dynamic thrust, push or throw

4. Eccentric-only movements, such as safe catching techniques for muscle control and stability

5. Concentric and eccentric movements, such as throw and catch and similar repetitive variations, such as pushing a ball back and forth against a wall

6. Explosive power movements (tests) with maximum recovery

Overview

1-2: Ensuring effective movement control, stability and body posture are pre-requisites in medicine ball training. This assists in maximizing future performance by making the movement more efficient and integrative by allowing the muscles and nervous system to adapt. Appropriate training creates chemical changes, which advance the capacity to do both central nervous system work and muscular endurance work under conditions of correct technique, before fatigue is reached.

3-6: When an athlete is focusing on maximal speed, muscle control and explosiveness (throws, thrusts and catches) with the ball, the central nervous system is highly taxed, requiring recovery periods of up to 3 minutes or more between sets so you are fresh. Also a minimum 48-72-hour recovery period between training is necessary to allow for proper recovery from dynamic drills. This is very important to understand because the body responds much differently to this type of training stimulus and requires sufficient recovery time even though you may not feel this way. This happens because it's more of a neural (or neuromuscular) training demand that fatigues the central nervous system and overloads muscles tissues, without you often knowing or feeling it. This occurs because of the dynamic requirements placed on the body with higher intensity power training, including drills referred to as plyometrics.

Plyometrics

Plyometric drills refer to any exercise where the muscle is contracted eccentrically, then immediately concentrically. In other words, the muscle is pre-stretched (loaded) before it is contracted, often referred to as a stretch-shortening cycle. A good example of the upper body undergoing plyometrics is performing a push-up with a clap. Your arm muscle is elongated and loaded by the downward force of your body, then immediately you must contract the muscle to push yourself back up explosively, before clapping, landing and repeating the action without loss of form or speed. Plyometrics are seen as an important developmental phase associated with improving all sporting actions involving explosive power, such as running, jumping and throwing.

Four basic concepts in the understanding of plyometric training:

1. Placing muscles under pre-stretch and working from eccentric to concentric incorporates reflexive responses

2. The rate of the stretch is more important than the length or magnitude of the stretch. Hence, quick pre-stretch movements are desired over longer ones

3. Activities promote the use of proper form, and improve balance, coordination, technique, skill, and body and functional awareness

4. Training with a pre-stretch and activation of neuromuscular components improves the efficiency of neural actions and muscular performance

In order to realize the potential of plyometric training, the stretch-shortening cycle must be invoked. This requires careful attention to the technique used during each drill or exercise. Training with a pre-stretch and activation of neuromuscular components improves the efficiency of neural actions and muscular performance. Once speed or power is reduced or fatigue sets in, the exercise needs to be stopped and recovery implemented. This is why establishing a strong core strength foundation or endurance through general strength is so important as a prerequisite to power or plyometric training.

Plyometric Medicine Ball Sports Training

Plyometrics are hopping, skipping, jumping and bounding exercises that train an athlete's neuromuscular system to fire quickly and gain explosiveness. Training with a pre-stretch and activation of neuromuscular components improves the efficiency of neural actions and muscular performance. Plyometric training seeks to enhance the explosive reaction of the individual through powerful muscular contractions as a result of rapid eccentric contractions. Simply, this means quick pre-stretch movements are desired over longer, slower movements.

When using a medicine ball, you can overload the muscle tissues in the exact pattern of movement you will use in a sport environment. Certain medicine ball exercises can also be used as part of a plyometric training program to develop explosive movements. With higher-than-normal forces placed on the musculoskeletal system during these exercises, it is important for the athlete to have a good, sound base of general strength and endurance. The coach should assess the athlete to determine if he/she has an adequate strength basis for participation. This pre-test can determine an athlete's limitations in flexibility, range of motion, posture, balance and stability, strength and coordination during the execution of exercises. How quickly an athlete loses form and technique is generally a good indication of any athlete's ability level, which can give you a idea of the basic level to start and progress from.

Quality and Intensity of Movement

As an athlete, power training effectively teaches you how to recruit the muscles that you've worked so hard to build. In medicine ball training, speed of movement is related to intensity. Even though the medicine ball is a light training implement, when thrown or caught, it produces large tissue tensions that can correlate to high-resistance training, such as weight training. With any exercise, the higher the intensity, the fewer repetitions (or time on task) should be performed. If you do too many repetitions with an intense exercise, the quality of the movement pattern will break down. As a result, the athlete is more likely to injure joint structures, muscle and connective tissue.

Essentially, all sets should never last longer than 6-10 seconds or include too many repetitions of explosive continuous power exercise, because the anaerobic energy system often becomes exhausted. In other cases, individual thrusts or throws across to a partner may involve less than a 1 second explosion followed by a recovery ratio of up to 5 or 10 seconds between throws, between partners, meaning the set may last for up to 60 seconds even though only 6 seconds of effort is applied (depending on the drill). Adapt accordingly, always focusing on quality of movement.

Recovery

Generally, the faster the movement of the exercise and the higher the intensity, then the greater the involvement is from the central nervous system (CNS). The greater this involvement, the more recovery time the athlete needs. In performing multi-joint exercises at high speeds, increased length of rest periods of up to 3 minutes or more are required to allow the CNS to recover. If the athlete is not recovering properly, he will find a breakdown in the movement pattern, reducing the quality of motor learning and overall power development.

In addition, the higher the skill level of the movement pattern, the longer the rest period should be. Simply put, the more mental activity there is, the more likely the person is to fatigue and not perform the movement pattern with precision. So, in order to ensure adequate recovery, your rest period must be long enough so that the athlete can perform the movement pattern you're trying to train him in with quality, intensity and accuracy each time.

Medicine Ball Sizes

The weight of the medicine ball will depend on the athlete's training age, training purpose and sport. Having a selection of sizes available will enable you to modify intensity accordingly for strength, speed or power applications.

Due to high neuromuscular involvement, especially among neutralizer and stabilizer muscles and joints, it is possible to reach muscle failure without showing any of the usual signs of physiological failure. For this reason, do not rely solely on conventional measures of fatigue to measure an athlete's recovery rate, but instead also on one's speed and quality of movement.
Teaching activities that are suitable for the athlete's level of development is essential. Stressing a progression from the simple to more difficult exercises enables the coach to pay greater attention to the athletes' physical ability to perform the activity. Commence with general whole body activities, and as the athlete develops, move to skills requiring finer motor control through the six developmental stages. Once general skills are acquired, your athlete will find it easier to pick up new techniques.

Rubber Medicine Ball Size	Training Purpose	Rest Periods Between Sets
1-2kg	• Strength endurance • Sport-specific power throws	• 60–120 seconds • 180 or more seconds
3-4kg	• Strength endurance • Sport-specific power • 3kg maximum size for kids 8-12 years old • 4kg maximum size for teens 13-17 years old	• 30–60 seconds • 180 seconds or more
5-6kg	• Core strength, such as abdominal work and push ups • Explosive power for senior athletes • Adult athletes only	• 30–60 seconds • 180 seconds or more

Technique and Safety

- Controlling the muscular function of the abdominal muscles and maintaining a deep breathing pattern is central to all activities. It is a prerequisite for maximizing force application and reducing the risk of injury.

- Because the body adapts to imposed demands, we tend to be strong in support on the legs, but relatively weak in support in the arms. Therefore, it is important to progressively strengthen the wrist, elbow and shoulder joints, starting with isolated movements and deep, controlled breathing patterns before moving onto a range of movement drills.

- Always progress exercises using a light ball at a slow to moderate pace. Firstly, to increase body awareness; secondly, to assess motor coordination; thirdly, to increase muscle and joint strength before adapting to a heavier ball.

- To reduce eccentric loads on the muscles and joints, always allow the ball to bounce before catching or receiving it. Minimize eccentric (catching) loads to close range at controlled speeds for muscle and neural adaptations before progressing. Apply low loads only after a minimum of 4 weeks of base training.

- Always train under the guidance of a qualified fitness professional or coach to ensure that correct technique is maintained and appropriate rest and recovery periods are adhered to.

Warm-up and Coordination Drills

Exercises are performed at a slow to moderate pace for 10 to 30 seconds to warm up the various muscle groups for the more dynamic tasks that lie ahead.

1. Around the Body

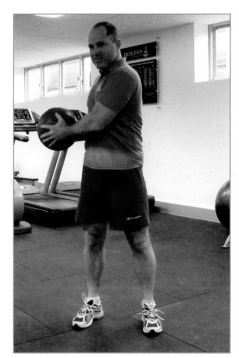 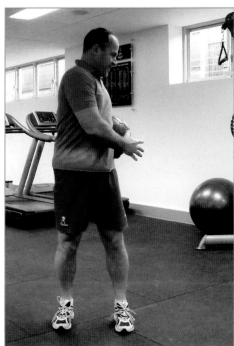

Across body   *Loop around back*

Description
- Rotate a medicine ball around the body in clockwise and anti-clockwise directions in a standing position. Also do this while walking and/or jogging forward or backwards.

2. Figure 8s (Between the Legs)

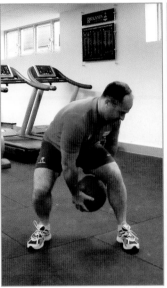

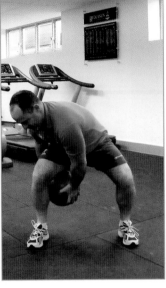

Description
- Stand in a wide squat position and loop a medicine ball in and out of your legs in a Figure 8 movement pattern.

Figure 8s

Back, around and through the legs

3. Knee-ups

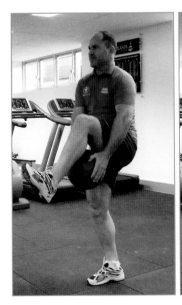

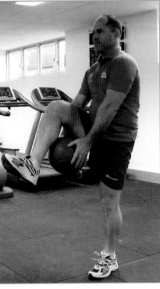

Description
- Holding a medicine ball in your left hand, raise your right knee high, scooping the medicine ball underneath the raised leg and catching the ball in your right hand. Repeat the sequence by raising your left leg while maintaining an upright body position.

Under left leg

Under right leg

4. Chest Pass

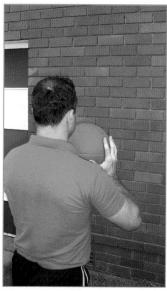
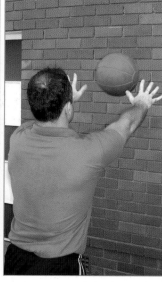

Start

Push to wall and catch

Description
- Stand 1-2 meters from a solid, concrete wall. Push and catch a light medicine ball against the wall in a fluid motion, performing chest passes for a set amount of time. Start slow and gradually build up to a moderate pace only.

5. Controlled Squat

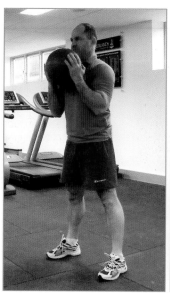
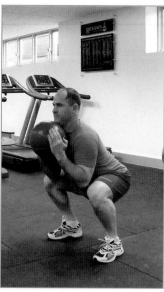

Start

Mid-point

Description
- Stand with your feet shoulder-width apart and a medicine ball held on your chest. Slowly lower your body by bending your knees until at a 90-degree angle, then rise upward.

Note: Extend the arms when rising to perform a squat, push-press.

Strength and Power Drills

6. Close-grip Push-ups

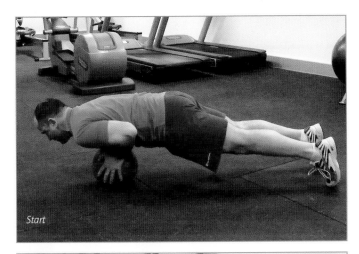

Start

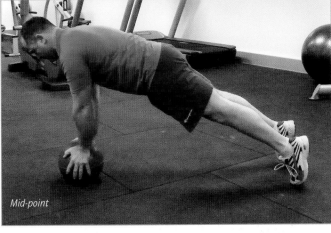

Mid-point

Description

- Resting on your toes, lie on a medicine ball at chest level and place both hands on the side of ball with your fingers pointing down and thumbs facing forward
- Brace the abdominal muscles and keep your posture straight to avoid arching the lower back
- Maintain your shoulders over the ball to ensure good alignment
- While breathing out, extend the arms and raise the body up
- Breathe in and lower the body onto the medicine ball
- Keep your head in a neutral position aligned with the body at all times for the development of good posture and technique

Variation:
- Push-ups on knees

7. Collins Push-ups

Description
- Start in the front support position with your hands placed shoulder-width apart with one hand on the medicine ball
- Brace the abdominal muscles and keep your posture straight to avoid arching the lower back
- Maintain your shoulder over the ball to ensure good alignment
- While breathing out, extend the arms and raise the body up
- Breathe in and lower the body until the rear of the upper arm (triceps) is in alignment with the body at a slight angle
- Keep the head in neutral position aligned with body at all times for the development of good posture and technique
- Repeat the drill with the opposite hand on the medicine ball

Variations
- Collins push-up roll
- Power cross

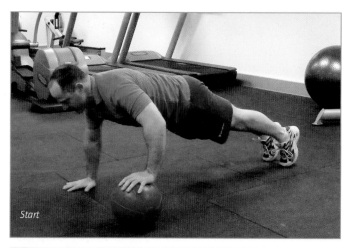

Start

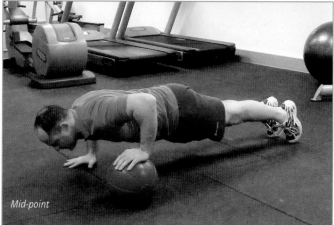

Mid-point

8. Collins Kneeling Push-up Roll

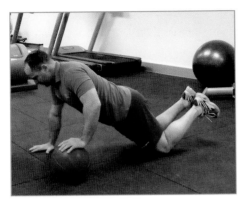

1. Start

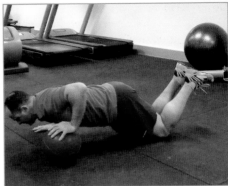

2. Mid-point

Description

- Start in the front support position with your hands placed shoulder-width apart with one hand on the medicine ball
- Brace the abdominal muscles and keep your posture straight to avoid arching the lower back
- Keep your shoulder over the ball to ensure good alignment
- Breathe in and lower the body until the rear of the upper arm (triceps) is in alignment with the body at a slight angle

3. Roll ball across

- While breathing out, extend the arms and raise the body up.
- As you return to the arm extension position, roll the medicine ball across the floor to the other hand
- Repeat the push-up action on the opposite side
- Keep your head in a neutral position aligned with body at all times for the development of good posture and technique

Variations

- Perform the drill in front support position on your toes
- Power cross

9. Power Push-ups

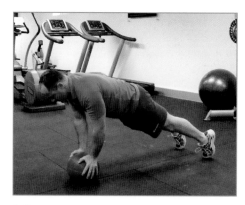

1. Start

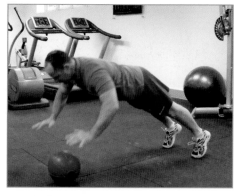

2. Push-off

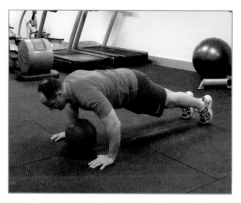

3. Land and absorb

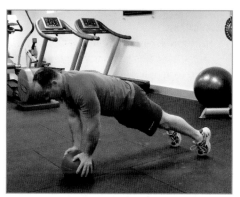

4. Explode back up onto ball

Description
- Begin in push-up position with your hands on the medicine ball, fingers facing down and thumbs forward
- Brace the abdominal muscles and keep your posture straight to avoid arching the lower back
- Quickly remove your hands from the medicine ball and drop down
- Land on the ground with both hands on either side of the medicine ball, more than shoulder-width apart
- Immediately react and push up by extending the elbows and placing your hands back on top of the medicine ball
- Repeat the action for set amount of repetitions. If form is lost, stop the exercise and recover
- Maintain good body posture at all times as quality of movement is desired over quantity

10. Power Cross

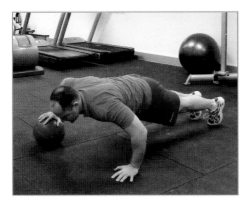

1. Start

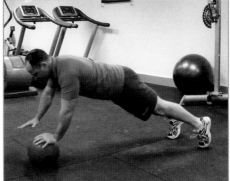

2. Mid-point cross-over

Description

- Begin in push-up position with one hand on the medicine ball and elbows bent
- Brace your abdominal muscles and keep your posture straight to avoid arching the lower back
- Explode up and across by extending the elbows
- Switch your hands on the ball and take the opposite hand out to the side to once again move into push-up position
- Quickly remove your hands from the medicine ball and drop down
- Immediately react and repeat the action across to the opposite side again for a set number of repetitions
- Maintain good body posture at all times as quality of movement is desired over quantity

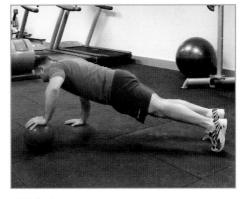

3. End-point

11. Lunge with Rotation Across the Body

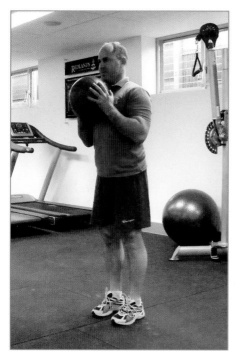
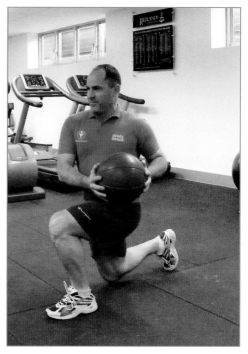

Start   Mid-point

Description
- Stand with your feet together holding the medicine ball in both hands at chest height
- Brace the abdominal muscles and keep your posture straight to avoid arching the lower back
- Step forward into in a lunge position with your right leg forward and left leg back (as shown), lowering the rear knee toward he ground without touching. At the same time, twist the medicine ball across your body over the right leg
- Ensure the hips are held square and the eyes are looking forward at all times to maintain good posture
- Lunge forward with the left leg and repeat the exercise by twisting the medicine ball across the left leg

Variations
- Lunge forward and then return back and repeat with the opposite leg
- Jump and land in lunge position on the spot (advanced athletes only)

12. Kick-ups

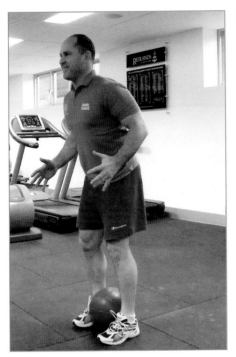

Start

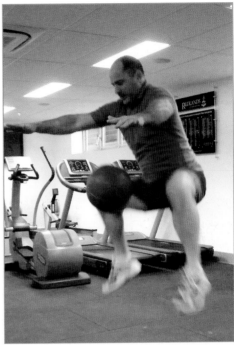

Mid-point

Description

- Stand tall with a medicine ball positioned between your feet and pressure placed against the ball
- In one motion, swing the arms forward and drive your knees and feet up with the medicine ball into the air
- Catch the ball in the air with your hands and land on the ground in strong body position – bending the knees to absorb the shock
- Return to the starting position and repeat

Variation

- Kick the ball up behind the body with a hamstring drive

13. Scoop Release

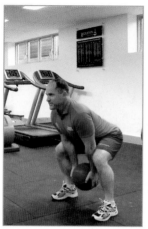

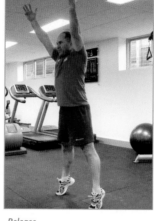

Mid-point   *Release*

Description
- Ensure a clear open space is available
- Stand with your feet shoulder-width apart and a medicine ball held in both hands, extended down at waist height in front of the body
- Brace your abdominal muscles and keep your posture straight to avoid arching the lower back
- Initiate the movement by bending your legs and squatting down until the legs are bent at a 90-degree angle, then power up, extending the legs and scooping the arms upward with the medicine ball forward and away from the body
- Upon release, walk, jog or sprint forward to retrieve the ball

Variation
- Scooping the ball overhead backwards

14. Power Throwdowns

Start

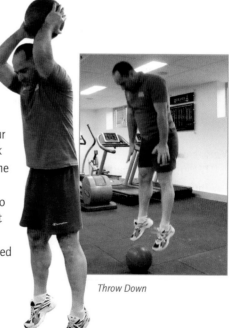

Description
- Stand with your feet parallel and the knees slightly bent
- Holding a medicine ball in your hands, extend the arms above your head
- Brace the abdominal muscles and keep your posture straight to avoid arching the lower back
- Jump up as you forcefully thrust the medicine ball to the ground in front of the body
- Land with control by bending the knees to absorb the shock. Catch the ball on the first bounce
- Repeat the drill according to prescribed repetitions

Throw Down

15. Triceps Thrust

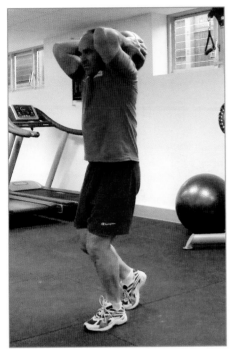
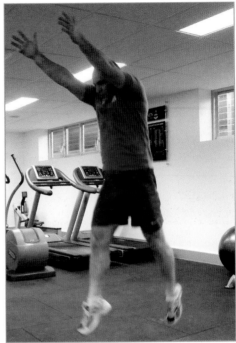

Start

Thrust Forward

Description
- Ensure a clear open space is available
- Stand with your feet together and the medicine ball overhead
- Hold the medicine ball with both hands, arms only slightly bent
- Brace the abdominal muscles and keep your posture straight to avoid arching the lower back
- Step forward and extend arms rapidly, releasing the medicine ball across the open area
- Land in lunge position and walk or jog forward to retrieve the medicine ball
- Maintain good body posture at all times as quality of movement is preferred over quantity

Variations
- Triceps thrust to partner – allow ball to bounce before catching
- Thrust against solid concrete wall 5-10 meters away – allow the ball to bounce before catching

Abdominal Region

The abdominal muscles support the trunk of your body, allow movement, and hold organs in place by regulating abdominal pressure. The abdominal muscles are made up of four different muscle groups, all with their own duties. Those four groups are the transversus abdominis, the rectus abdominis, the external oblique, and the internal oblique. The abdominal medicine ball exercises will help strengthen your lower, upper and oblique abdominal muscles. Many of these moves are power-based exercises involving catching and throwing using the arms and require good core strength of the upper body region.

To ensure personal safety, the following points should be noted:
- Brace the abdominal muscles to support the lower back
- Complete throws with full extension of the arms
- Focus on quality of movement and do not sacrifice control for distance
- When picking up a medicine ball, ensure the knees are bent and the back is kept straight
- Prior to catching a medicine ball, if required, keep your arms extended with hands close together; eyes on the ball; reach out to meet the ball prior to making contact and do not attempt to catch balls thrown wildly

16. Toe Touches

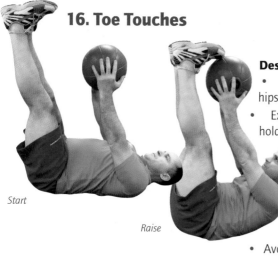

Start

Raise

Description
- Lie on your back with your legs raised from the hips at 90 degrees and slightly bent
- Extend your arms up above the eye-line while holding the medicine ball
- While breathing out, raise the shoulders off the ground and reach the medicine ball up toward your feet, then lower
- Avoid swinging your legs or creating a hip angle beyond 90 degrees due to the stress placed on the lower back
- Avoid leading the exercise with your chin. Use your abdominal muscles to drive the medicine ball in your hands up
- Repeat for the desired number of repetitions with good form

Variation
- Place your feet on the ground, knees bent. Raise the ball up to a similar position in a sit-up motion.

17. Overhead Toe Touches

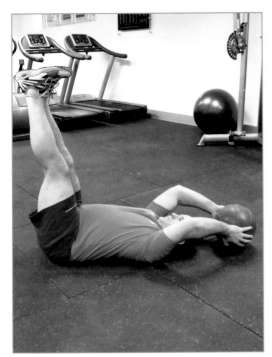

Start

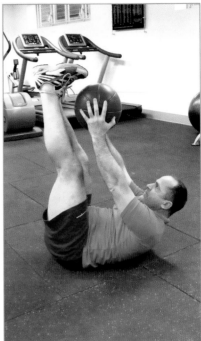

Raise

Descriptions
- Lie on your back with your legs raised from the hips at 90 degrees and slightly bent
- Extend your arms overhead holding medicine ball off the ground
- Brace abdominal muscles and keep posture straight to avoid arching the lower back
- While breathing out, initiate abdominal contractions while raising the medicine ball off the ground and reaching up toward feet, then lower in a controlled eccentric motion.
- Avoid swinging your legs or taking the hip angle beyond 90 degrees due to the stress placed on the lower back
- Avoid leading the exercise with your chin; use the abdominal muscles to drive the medicine ball in your hands up
- Repeat for the desired number of repetitions with good form

Variation
- Start with your legs extended and on the ground, then raise your arms and legs simultaneously.

18. Rotary Twist

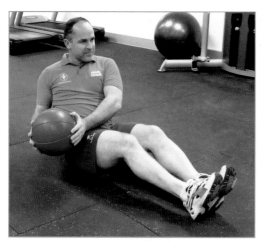

Right side

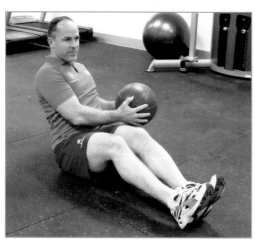

Left side

Description
- Sit back at a 45 to 60-degree angle from the hips and brace your abdominal muscles
- Avoid rounding the back; keep the spine in neutral position
- Extend your arms forward, slightly bent, while holding the medicine ball
- Maintaining a strong abdominal brace, slowly take the medicine ball across to the left knee then back across to the right knee
- Work only between the outside of each knee
- This exercise places a demand on the isometric abdominal brace being held by working the medicine ball at different angles

Variations
- Concentric-only thrusts up to partner (standing) who rolls the ball back
- Eccentric catch-only from partner (standing) – you roll the ball back
- Eccentric followed by concentric thrust with partner (standing)
- Eccentric followed by concentric thrust with partner (sitting)
- Continuous catch and throws against the wall

19. Abdominal Oblique Crossover

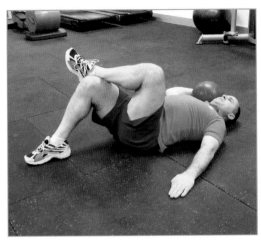

Start

Description
- Lie on your back with:
  - Left leg bent and left foot resting on right thigh
  - Medicine ball resting on the right shoulder against the head and gripped by a hand
- Raise the right elbow across to the left knee, then lower
- Repeat for a set number of repetitions
- Repeat the exercise with the right leg bent and the medicine ball on the left shoulder

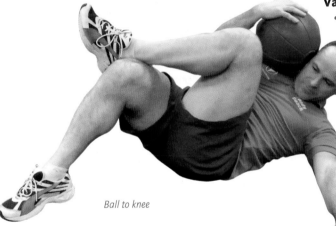

Ball to knee

Variation
- Start with the opposite leg straight, with shoulder against the medicine ball and raised off the ground. At the same time, bring your knee into your chest as your shoulder rises and the medicine ball crosses over toward the knee, then return back to starting position. Repeat.

20. Rotary thrust to wall

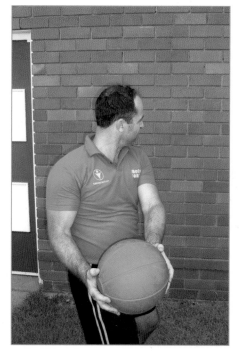

Start

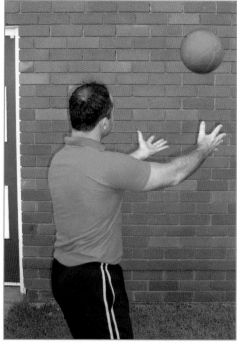

Thrust to wall, then catch

Description
- Stand in a lateral position with your feet hip-width apart, holding a medicine ball with both hands. Keep your arms slightly bent approximately 3-5 meters from a solid concrete wall
- Swing the ball over to the right hip and then forcefully rotate the ball forward across your body and release it toward the wall
- Initiate the forward thrust of the medicine ball, using your feet, hips, abdominal muscle rotation and arms
- Gently brace the abdominal muscles and allow your feet to pivot as your hips turn
- Stand close to the wall and catch
- Repeat the drill on the opposite side

Variations
- Allow the ball to bounce once off the wall before catching and repeating the movement
- Perform in a seated position on the ground
- Lunge cross thrusts

Partner Drills – Upper Body

21. Front Support Power Push

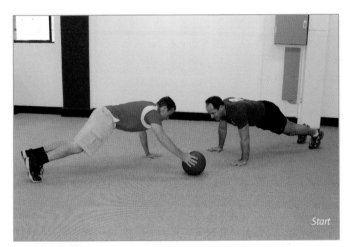

Start

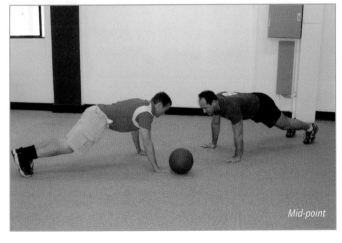

Mid-point

Description

- Start in front support position 1-2 meters from partner, head-to-head
- Brace the abdominal muscles and keep your posture straight to avoid arching the lower back
- Partner A places the medicine ball in front of your right hand
- Partner A pushes the medicine ball across to Partner B while maintaining a strong core position of the body
- Partner B traps the ball and pushes it back to Partner A
- Maintain continuous motion forward and backward
- Vary angles pushed toward left hand, right hand, middle and wide
- Maintain good body posture at all times as quality of movement is preferred over quantity

Variations
- Increase or decrease distance between partners
- Perform for a set amount of time
- Vary angles, including the inside and outside hand position

185

22. Plyometric Push-ups

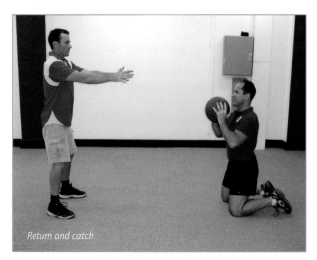

Return and catch

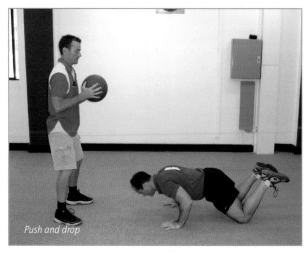

Push and drop

Description

- Kneel on the ground holding a medicine ball on your chest
- Partners stand 3-10 meters away ready to catch and return the ball using the following variations:
- Concentric medicine ball push to eccentric body weight landing in front support position. The ball is rolled back by the partner
- Concentric medicine ball push to eccentric body weight landing in front support position followed directly with a concentric explosion back up to kneeling position. Ball is rolled back by the partner
- Concentric medicine ball push to eccentric body weight landing in front support position followed directly with a concentric explosion back up to kneeling position to catch a ball (eccentrically) thrown by a partner. Rest before repeating

- Repeat concentric and eccentric push and catch in a continuous motion for a set amount of repetitions or time
- Increase the weight of the medicine ball to increase the intensity
- **Advanced:** Both partners knee on the ground 3-10 meters apart. Start slow and gradually increase speed without loss of form – quality over quantity.

23. Lateral Shuffle Pass

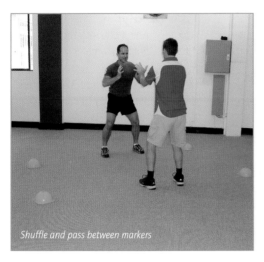
Shuffle and pass between markers

Description
- Draw two parallel lines 2-5 meters apart and 10 meters long
- Athletes face each other, with one holding a medicine ball at chest height
- Brace the abdominal muscles and keep your posture straight to avoid arching the lower back
- Athletes perform a chest pass with the medicine ball back and forth while moving laterally along the lines
- Ensure the passes are maintained at chest height. Also ensure good posture and technique

Variations
- Start with a very light medicine ball and perfect the movement before adding a higher load.
- One athlete stands still while the other athlete maneuvers along the line when the ball is passed to catch and return

24. 30-second Pick-up

Description
- One athlete stands approximately 5 meters from Partner B who is holding a medicine ball
- On the word "go," Partner A throws the medicine ball in any direction
- Partner B has to chase, pick up and throw the ball back to Partner A
- Partner A repeats throws for Partner B for 30 seconds to help improve fitness levels

Variations
- Use a light medicine ball to start with and throw in multiple directions
- Use 10 to 60-second variations

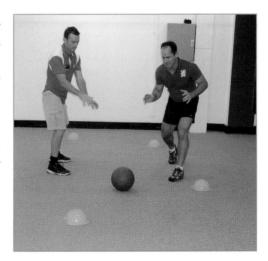
Chase, pick-up and return for up to 30 seconds

25. Leg Curls

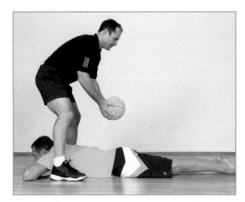
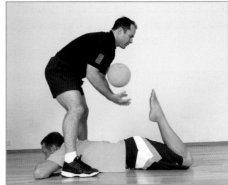

Start   *Overhead Thrust*

Description
- Partner A lies on his stomach with his hands under his chin, feet together and toes pointed
- Partner B stands at shoulder level facing Partner A's feet, holding a medicine ball in his hands in a semi-squat position
- Partner B rolls the ball down the back of Partner A's legs toward his feet. As the ball reaches toward the calves, Partner A curls his legs and kicks the medicine ball back up to Partner B by flexing the knees
- Partner B holds his hands up ready to catch the ball, whichever way it travels from the kick, then returns to the starting position and repeats the drill

Notes:
- If both legs are even in strength, the ball should return straight when curled back. An imbalance in leg strength will lead to the ball being kicked to the side
- Partner B should be conscious at all times with both hands raised ready to catch the medicine ball. If Partner A has a strong kick, Partner B may need to move farther away from Partner A for a more effective catch

Body Coach® Education, Training & Products

Join The Body Coach® Paul Collins, international author and strength and conditioning coach, and his team of experts in the Fastfeet® Speed for Sport Training clinics, workshops, camps, seminars and coaching for all sports

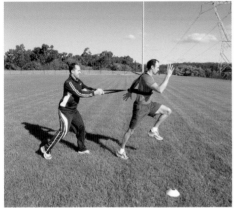 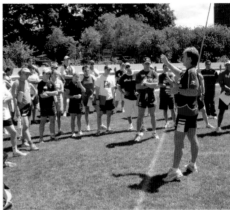

Paul Collins and Ron Palmer presenting a Speed for Sport Coaching Seminar

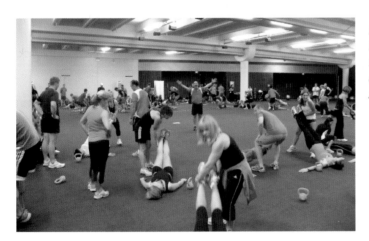

Paul Collins presenting Kettlebell Training at the International Filex Fitness conference, Sydney, Australia

For more details and products, visit the following websites:
www.thebodycoach.com
www.bodycoach.com.au
www.fastfeet.com.au

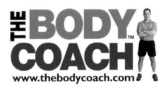

Kettlebell Training Index

Photo & Illustration Credits:

Cover Photo: © Damir Spanic/iStockphoto LP
Cover Design: Sabine Groten
Photos: Paul Collins